THE
ARCHIPELAGO OF
CONSCIOUSNESS

THE
ARCHIPELAGO OF CONSCIOUSNESS

The Invisible Sovereignty of Life

Mauro Maldonato

Translated by
Mark Weir

sussex
ACADEMIC
PRESS
Brighton • Chicago • Toronto

First published in English translation, 2015, by
SUSSEX ACADEMIC PRESS
PO Box 139
Eastbourne BN24 9BP

and in the United States of America by
SUSSEX ACADEMIC PRESS
Independent Publishers Group
814 N. Franklin Street, Chicago, IL 60610

and in Canada by
SUSSEX ACADEMIC PRESS (CANADA)
24 Ranee Avenue, Toronto, Ontario, M6A 1M6

British Library Cataloguing in Publication Data
A CIP catalogue record for this book is available from the British Library.

Library of Congress Cataloging-in-Publication Data
Maldonato, Mauro.
[Arcipelago della coscienza]
The archipelago of consciousness : the invisible sovereignty of life /
   Mauro Maldonato.
    pages   cm
Includes bibliographical references and index.
ISBN 978-1-84519-712-4 (pb : alk. paper)
1. Consciousness. 2. Neuropsychology. I. Title.
BF311.M19813 2015
152—dc23
                                                                    2014043297

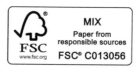

Typeset and designed by Sussex Academic Press, Brighton & Eastbourne.
Printed by TJ International, Padstow, Cornwall.

CONTENTS

Man and the Sea

Free man, you will always cherish the sea!
The sea is your mirror; you contemplate your soul
In the infinite unrolling of its billows;
Your mind is an abyss that is no less bitter.
You like to plunge into the bosom of your image;
You embrace it with eyes and arms, and your heart
Is distracted at times from its own clamoring
By the sound of this plaint, wild and untamable.
Both of you are gloomy and reticent:
Man, no one has sounded the depths of your being;
O Sea, no person knows your most hidden riches,
So zealously do you keep your secrets!
Yet for countless ages you have fought each other
Without pity, without remorse,
So fiercely do you love carnage and death,
O eternal fighters, implacable brothers!

CHARLES BAUDELAIRE

Dark things tend towards clarity (. . .).

EUGENIO MONTALE

Everyone carries a shadow,
and the less it is embodied in the individual's conscious life,
the blacker and denser it is.

CARL GUSTAV JUNG

PROLOGUE

The rush of our thought forward through its fringes is the everlasting peculiarity of its life. We realize this life as something always off its balance, something in transition, something that shoots out of a darkness through a dawn into a brightness that we feel to be the dawn fulfilled.

WILLIAM JAMES

And going on, we come to things like evil, and beauty, and hope . . .
Which end is nearer to God, if I may use a religious metaphor, beauty and hope, or the fundamental laws? I think that the right way, of course, is to say that what we have to look at is the whole structural interconnection of the thing; and that all the sciences, and not just the sciences but all the efforts of intellectual kinds, are an endeavor to see the connections of the hierarchies, to connect beauty to history, to connect history to man's psychology, man's psychology to the working of the brain, the brain to the neural impulse, the neural impulse to the chemistry, and so forth, up and down, both ways. And today we cannot, and it is no use making believe that we can, draw carefully a line all the way from one end of this thing to the other, because we have only just begun to see that there is this relative hierarchy. And I do not think either end is nearer to God.

RICHARD FEYNMAN

The earth went on quaking for a long time, millions of years ago in north-eastern Tanzania. An enormous column of smoke and ashes rose up to block out the sun; driven by the wind, it deposited itself over everything in a range of thousands of kilometres. While animals of all species sought refuge as best they could, some *australopiths* found safety by plunging down into the dense rain forest. But it was not long before they were on the move again. Skirting round the edge of the Rift Valley, they turned their backs on the Ngorongoro plateau and the majestic Lengai, the Mountain of God venerated by the Masai. Perhaps this was how the adventure of the human race began. On that long journey the young hominids would have learned to live in a group, to explore new territories and map them, to subjugate nature by means of husbandry and agriculture. Above all they invented language, after communicating for so long merely by grunts and vague intimations. Then, not long after instinct and learning, self-consciousness made its appearance, and with it the ability to reflect on one's own behaviour and immediate environment. It was in fact consciousness that fostered the impatient need to know, driving man towards unknown lands and to the far ends of the earth. Soon he began to contemplate the heavens and the meaning of things, sensing mystery and fascination. Who knows if, in the starry nights or witnessing the pure tracts of dawn, he did not feel overawed at the spectacle of the universe, and perhaps catch a glimpse of that nature that transcends and dominates us? Amazement at the incommensurable diversity of the world did not merely attenuate its brutality: it also induced him to penetrate ever more deeply into the surprising mystery of life. His own self image reflected in others, his thought processes and all the other sensations he experienced within himself formed his mind, setting in motion the selection of the best models of behaviour.

But how, and above all when, did all this begin? No one can say. The first forms of life appeared on earth three billion years ago and perhaps more. It was not until a billion years later that life's first building blocks began to come together: proteins and whatever else was necessary for survival and reproduction. How is it possible that simple blobs of jelly, dispersed in the primordial waters, can have generated life forms able to develop and reproduce, culminating in that inconceivable experiment of intelligent life that resisted the ice ages and the planet's geological mutations? We would require a minutely detailed natural history in order to grasp what an extraordinary innovation the emergence of "mind" was in the evolution of the human race, and above all to clarify the scope of those behavioural models which rewarded the individuals who were best able to respond to the unforeseeable events that took place around them and to cater for their own essential requisites.

We have to admit that it is extremely difficult to imagine how the mind evolved from the inflexible laws of matter. Was it a fortuitous occurrence in the course of evolution, whose meaning is not clear to us, or was there something else? And how are we to account for the progressive increase in the human brain's complexity? However we look at the circumstances that have led to our present state, the progress has been anything but linear. We do not even know whether man, in his present state, represents the crowning achievement for the species. We only know that the integration of entities that were previously separate is a constant feature of our universe. Fundamentally the (relative) certainty that our fellow men are endowed like us with consciousness is merely based on the similarity of our brains. This is really as far as our certainties go. What will never be in doubt is that the genesis of *thinking matter* is the most surprising event of all in evolution. Is there not something miraculous in the fact that molecules which are so different from one another should have come together to form a being that is conscious of himself and of the world? When compared with the slowness of the physical and chemical processes governing matter, intelligent life really does seem to be something of an exception.

For over a century now, scientists working in various disciplines all over the world have been trying to throw light on the secrets of the brain. But the better we become at tracing its labyrinths, explaining its mechanisms and mapping its geography, the more arduous is the task of explaining it. The nature, plasticity and unrepeatability of the brain's organization now appear much more dynamic and complex than anything we had ever suspected. To insist that the basis and substance of life is to be sought in simple matter, with all the rest being considered as merely accessory, risks leading the discussion into an impasse. Not only would a concept like "human liberty" be nonsensical; it would be like reducing Michelangelo's *Pietà* to the marble it is made from.

So what does lie behind thought processes, feelings, consciousness and the highest activities of the human mind? There can be no doubt about it: every mental event, even the most abstract, is correlated to events in the brain. Just as there is no question that lesions of specific areas of the brain cause loss of, or a deficit in, some of the mental faculties which are correlated to those areas. Besides, each specific area is inevitably involved both in the vital functions (acting, breathing, walking and so on) and in mental activities (remembering, dreaming, thinking), which only partially involve motor action. Moreover, not all mental activities can be easily located. For example, many faculties which are essential to survival, like memory, are based both in the cortex and in the subcortex. Other more general and abstract faculties – decision making, reasoning, judging – which are correlated to metabolic variations in the limbic and prefrontal areas, are even more difficult to locate. Even our relations with other human beings, like the elaboration of sensorial sources and the relative behavioural responses, appear to be mediated by processes scattered across the brain; specific areas become expert so that they can 'flexibilize' the inborn predispositions in the interests of a progressive, albeit relative, emancipation of the organism's behaviour patterns from environmental constrictions.

If this is the case, why is the materialistic viewpoint, even in its most rational and responsible guise, unable to determine what is taking place in the brain, bogged down as it is in unresolvable aporias. The etymology is complex, but "perplexity" is a good starting point. The materialistic viewpoint fails to convince because it is not able to describe the complexity of the brain; it presents an image which is too simplistic and static to provide an insight into the brain's extraordinary fundamental mechanisms.

The specious present

Surely the exceptional nature of consciousness has never been more effectively evoked than in Proust's recollections of *madeleines*. The echo of a far-off sensation generates in Marcel a stunning sensorial kaleidoscope. Fragments of experience, relegated to the archives of his memory, are brought back to life. *Mnemosyne* does not merely rescue Marcel from a sense of guilt, from anxieties and the contingency of the present. The ecstatic recollection provides a release from the extreme struggle between life and death. It does away with the filter between past and present. It breaks the arrow of time. It bestows immortality on him. People die when they are no longer able to connect the beginning and the end. The banks of Acheron will have a long time to wait. Even Proust's initial tendency to melancholy is redeemed by his remarkable trip into the mystery of memory.

Although itself a small piece of matter, that little cake in the shape of a shell, tasting of lemon, enables us to enter into the spirit of the writer.

> (. . .) No sooner had the warm liquid, and the crumbs with it, touched my palate than a shudder ran through my whole body, and I stopped, intent upon the extraordinary changes that were taking place. An exquisite pleasure had invaded my senses, but individual, detached, with no suggestion of its origin. And at once the vicissitudes of life had become indifferent to me, its disasters innocuous, its brevity illusory—this new sensation having had on me the effect which love has of filling me with a precious essence; or rather this essence was not in me, it was myself. I had ceased now to feel mediocre, accidental, mortal. Whence could it have come to me, this all-powerful joy? I was conscious that it was connected with the taste of tea and cake, but that it infinitely transcended those savours, could not, indeed, be of the same nature as theirs. Whence did it come? What did it signify? How could I seize upon and define it? I drink a second mouthful, in which I find nothing more than in the first, a third, which gives me rather less than the second. It is time to stop; the potion is losing its magic. It is plain that the object of my quest, the truth, lies not in the cup but in myself. (Proust, 1922, p. 49)

What is this variation in levels of reality due to? How did Marcel's consciousness lead him into that archipelago of memories that made his inner world such an extraordinary theatre for experimentation? How can one account for that example of pure freedom when, in *Time regained*, the narrator comes face to face with his destiny precisely where he had sought to avoid it? When he stumbles on the uneven flagstones in the courtyard of the Guermantes residence, Marcel is overcome by an ecstatic, atemporal epiphany. Just when everything seemed to be lost, a new path suddenly opens up before him. Without even having taking a decision, he feels ready to set about the work of art for which he was convinced he lacked the talent. What is this inexplicable and surprising happiness? Where is the source of that joy and sense of strength that are so intense as to make even the idea of death indifferent to him? What subtle enigma is concealed behind all this? This happiness transforms him immediately into a being emancipated from the yoke of time. And it is of no importance that Marcel proved to be expert at building and shaping. What counts is how his memory erected subtle, inexplicable structures that gave rise to a new form of life. This recognition of memory both sought and found, this paradoxical "rendering present" of what is absent, reveals the full profundity of time, the intentional quality of memory and the way in which consciousness is affected by events. Just as the age of a tree is imprinted in the concentric circles of its trunk, so memory keeps a record of events, physical occurrences and not only.

Materialists believe that all of this can be traced back to the brain and, in an infinite regression, to the cell nucleus, chromosomes, and so on. Yet it is not as simple as this. Of course, the brain is the outcome of a rigid genetical coding: its functioning depends on the interaction of an unlimited range of neuronal connections that are constantly being manufactured, on its plasticity, and on the elaboration of ever new sensorial inferences. Nonetheless, however sophisticated it may be, no genetic programming would ever be able to connect up the billions and billions of neurons in intercommunicating networks used to carry out our sophisticated mental activities. These activities depend on interaction with the external environment. And it is this relationship, along with innumerable others, that decides which connections will survive and which perish. Some years ago Gerald M. Edelman put forward the fascinating theory that the higher cerebral functions and the anatomical/functional changes that come about at birth in every animal organism are the outcome of a harsh phylogenetic selection. During life in the womb a large-scale suppression of neurons takes place, followed at birth by the decimation of all the redundant connections. In fact the adult brain is the product of a massive restructuring which has eliminated the connections that are least active so as to reinforce the most active.

The ignorant neuron

The brain does not just decide how to interact with the environment, it also facilitates the structural coupling between sensorial data and neurons, freeing the latter from their original 'ignorance'. This is the key to its approach to the world in terms of creation and invention. How could the shifting geographies of such a huge number of neuronal territories ever be mechanically reproduced? The structure and functions of the brain are continually influenced by all sorts of unpredictable factors (sensorial poverty or richness, quality and intensity of perception) which condition its development and connections. This is an ancient process that had already begun in the first phases of hominization, when maternal care and cultural interaction gave a strong impulse to the growth of the neuronal connections in the brain. Without these dynamics it would have been quite impossible for language, that formidable regulating principle of thought and representation of reality, to develop. For it is language that provides the procedures for classifying, abstracting and transforming objects in concepts. Thanks to language, too, perceptions are turned into abstract values, generalizations and moral judgements. How does all this come about? Above all, what relationship is there between language and the brain? It seems quite likely that the development of the cortical areas involved in communication was a consequence of the increasing part these areas played in the (apparent) control over the world.

But what is it that gives form and order to the world? What recovers the data and, through the senses, interrogates the external phenomena? What are the grounds for the innumerable interactions between the individual areas, the exchange of sensorial traces and data among highly intricate neuronal networks, the constant re-elaboration of pre-existing information, the collaboration and competition between the cortical and subcortical structures? What biological algorithm can govern the effects of contingency and historical irreversibility, the action of non-linear processes, artistic creation, ethical systems or the scientific vision of the world? Surely only consciousness can fulfil this. Prior to being the premise for awareness, consciousness is living matter, indeed, a "living body". Our thoughts spring from the body, or rather from the brain, which is first and foremost body. Certainly, the cortex, the physical location of fantasy and our capacity for abstraction, plays a crucial role in our relational existence, but it is consciousness – "wider than the sky", as Emily Dickinson memorably characterised it – that is the most authentic expression of the complexity that matter has reached in the course of its evolution.

It is only our inability to recognise our biological and psychic existences as a single whole which nurtures old and new dichotomies and prompts us to give more credit to the ambiguous messages that come from the world around us than to ourselves. Only an ideology, or faith in a particular world view, can make us deny the existence of facts and things that go beyond the physical world. Materialism – meaning literally belief in the existence only of matter – does not explain reality. What objective forms of knowledge, what epistemology based on the brain, can provide me with information about the experiences of a being who is different from me? The more I distance my "self" from myself, to ensure the objectivity of my criteria and judgements, the more my perception of things becomes hazy. Even the hypothesis of the identity between mental and physical states begins to seem fallacious. For to maintain that a mental state *is* a physical state requires arguments that are more convincing than a mere understanding of the workings of the verb "to be". If we fail to get to grips with materialism's theoretical hypothesis, this will continue to be an obstacle on the path to a fruitful knowledge of consciousness.

We are a bit like mariners obliged to carry out repairs to their vessel while at sea, with only a few virtually useless tools to hand. We do not know if we will be able to construct a new *science of consciousness*, but there is no doubt that nothing will be as it was before. Relating consciousness to the body means recognising the unique complexity of the path nature has taken to date. But, even more crucially, it means admitting that the truly remarkable miracle of our universe is the existence of nature itself, that nature which we know is subject to the implacable laws of physics and chemistry. From the very start matter has been constituted in increasingly complex forms. In its formidable mutations it has learnt to assimilate and transmit information, to become an exceptional vehicle for the non-material, whether we are speaking of stars, galaxies or human beings. Matter decays and is transformed, is renewed and divides. On the contrary, information is constantly expanding, leaving its mark in basic aggregates of molecules, and above all generating an inconceivable increase of sense in the history of the universe. If we do not recognise all this, we are bound to remain trapped in the age-old dichotomy of matter and spirit.

From the neuron to consciousness

Among the many obstacles making it difficult for a science of consciousness to evolve, there is the dogma whereby science has to be objective. Maybe the time has come to give a different meaning to the objective–subjective relationship. As we shall see when we look at *qualia* – qualitative experiences which are elusive, private, immediate and not inference-based, that make us see things they way they appear to be –

making a strict distinction between the mind and consciousness has prevented the emergence of a common scientific perspective on the nature of conscious experience. On one hand are those who deny the existence of experiences that cannot be attributed to physical processes; and on the other, those who assert the existence of two irreconcilable realities: thought and matter (or at least, as the advocates of the dualism of properties claim, of mental events which are qualitatively different to the physical processes that determine them). We have to ask whether it is possible to study consciousness and its properties using the tools and methods of the natural sciences. But since the mind can only be studied if it is a physical substance, the answer must be affirmative. The natural world is physical and, therefore, accessible to all. For example, anyone possessing the appropriate instruments could ascertain that neutrinos travel faster than the speed of light. But no one can gain access to the universe of the mind because only the subject of the experiment can probe it. It is true that the neuronal structures of an organism can be scanned at the precise moment in which something is being experienced, but we shall never know the real meaning of that experience. When we describe states of the brain we are only describing the state of the neuron populations, not the qualitative experience or intentionality of the subject whose brain is being scanned. Intentional objects elude the biological models which refer to neurophysiological values in the brain (for example, an increase in the blood flow, metabolic variations, etc.) that can be instrumentally registered. Only once consciousness is naturalised can we break free from the paralysing interpretative dilemmas. And what does this naturalisation involve? Making sense of the nervous mechanisms of the intentionality and qualitative awareness which enable us to relate to our peers, to convey our desires and beliefs to them, and ultimately to understand what others are doing and why.

In the domain of the cognitive neurosciences a number of researchers are beginning to investigate the neural correlates of the elements embodied in our experience of the world, turning their backs on the sterile assumption that identified the mind with all things theoretical. In other words there is a growing awareness of the need for research, grounded in the premises of the neurosciences, which takes the body and its sensomotorial neural correlates as its prime object of enquiry. Our relationship with the world is mediated by the body and thus by the senses – our means of accessing the world. Until quite recently many neuroscientists were adamant that functions such as sensation, perception and the control of motor action were localised in precise areas of the cortex (sensations above all in the primary sensory areas; perception as the expression of associative areas; action generated by the motor areas linked to the activities of the frontal lobe). According to this palpably

"Victorian" neurophysiological model, the analysis of the external world merely consists in a flow of information passing from the sensorial cortex areas to the frontal motor areas, where it is integrated with the elaboration of the prefrontal cortex, site of processes involving judgement, choice and the higher functions of our relational life.

If it were possible to remedy the lazy reflexes we have inherited, current research programmes could perhaps be re-oriented so as to make the relationship between intentionality and cerebral processes (e.g. the red light that immediately makes us step on the brake pedal) less obscure, and above all throw light on the way in which an intentional state influences the external world. Obviously the questions concerning the relationship between seeing a colour and neuronal activity do not stop here. If, within certain limits, we are able to know whether a material object or a physical event really are as they appear to be, it is extremely difficult to know if a subjective experience is different to how it appears. The truth of an experience is on the surface; things reveal themselves on a surface but which speaks on behalf of a depth. There is no mental ontology which is independent of conscious experience. Denying the intentionality of consciousness on the grounds that only matter exists fails to clarify anything. How could the materialists ever hope to explain expectation and revelation, desire and nostalgia, courage and hope? Neither dualists nor materialists have adequately faced up to the problem of consciousness, for the former simply deny the existence of subjectivity, while the latter divide up reality into separate categories. Even if the mind is part of nature, so the dualist argument goes, this does not account for the whole of reality. True enough! But this tells us nothing about how the mind intervenes in a dynamic of cause and effect on physical entities. The physical world is anything but a self-contained structure; if it were self-sufficient, mental events would only be a superficial, and largely insignificant, effect of the brain.

This book sets out to show that consciousness is an original event generated by the interaction of different levels – neural infrastructures, qualitative-subjective experiences and functional units – that are logically inter-connected. Why do we speak of an *original bio-physical event* rather than an *emerging event*? Because the latter concept involves a number of ambiguities. In everyday discourse, the term "emergence" indicates the appearance of a new order of things from the interaction of the elements of a system: this phenomenon – present in both elementary and highly complex environments – cannot be inferred from the action of the individual components of the system. High levels of complexity make it difficult (if not impossible) to reduce a phenomenon to its elementary components. It is clear that one must exercise prudence when it comes to announcing the emergence of something new.

There is no doubt that studies in physics concerning chaotic phenomena and dynamic systems that deny equilibrium have added to our store of knowledge. However, this does not mean that concepts like emergence or auto-organization have enabled us to make significant progress in our understanding of elementary neuro-biological processes. And besides, the statement that consciousness must have emerged from auto-adaptive processes is like saying that an observed event has been mechanically produced by a 'lower-level' structure or that deterministic phenomena generate others that are not deterministic. Taken to its extreme consequences, emergence would be a sort of reductionism that is even more radical than its classic counterpart. In fact, whereas in classic reductionism the process of reduction was methodologically limited to nervous functions ordered according to a hierarchy, nowadays the process of reduction is ontologically extended to the whole range of phenomena, from the neuron to consciousness.

A constantly changing chimera

More than a century ago psychoanalysis set neurology and psychiatry an unprecedented challenge by revealing that the effects of the unconscious are more potent than those of consciousness, and that unconscious drives are constantly trying to surface in conscious life. Freud would often remark that psychological acts do not just float about in the air and that one day, perhaps not even so far off, the combined efforts of biologists and psychoanalysts would come up with a common explanation for psychic processes. Today, *mutatis mutandis*, the neurosciences are challenging psychoanalysis with experimental and clinical models that are clarifying the language of the neurons, the brain's plastic capacity, and other crucial aspects of the human mind.

Over the last fifty years a genuine revolution has taken place. The rapid development of methods of neuro-imaging (non-invasive techniques for investigating the cerebral functions in their functional version which show the brain's activity while we are performing an action, thinking, becoming emotional, and so on) and, above all, the ever closer matching of experimental and clinical data, have ushered in a new era of research, making progress that until recently was simply unimaginable. Nonetheless, the neurosciences are facing a number of questions that cannot be eluded. For example, how does the brain generate states of awareness? Do the activities of consciousness involve only limited zones of the brain or is it a global phenomenon in which the brain plays only a part, albeit a highly significant one? Or again, if consciousness were due to the activity of specific regions, would it involve the activity of specific types of neurons or a variety of anatomical substrata? In this case, which level would be correlated: the intracellular structures, the synapses, or specific neuronal stratifications? We shall not be able to make much progress until we can throw light on these questions.

Why should one write a book about consciousness? It is not difficult to reply: out of sheer wonder at the marvel of life. But also out of dissatisfaction with how the subject is currently being treated. It is time for a wide-ranging debate on this subject that goes far beyond the confines of the classic disciplines. The urge to come up with a single, uniform explanation for mental phenomena has made the discussion ambiguous and confused. Certainly, it is understandable that researchers should defend their own ideas, and even the terminology underpinning the identity of their particular disciplines, in science as in everyday life. But there can be no justification for refusing to engage in dialogue. Whoever sets out to investigate such demanding problems cannot shy away from critical exchanges, which have their use even when on-going dialogue proves to be impossible. On the terrain of research, the impossibility of a confrontation should derive from the importance of a subject or an issue, not from prejudices based on methodology or doctrine, or on a dogmatic insistence on certain tenets, which are all the more intolerable when we are dealing with a topic as daunting as consciousness.

In the debate on consciousness many concepts have come to seem inadequate. They should now perhaps be left to their own fate, at least those which are most patently inadequate. We are confronted with a scientific and cultural watershed. Nobody can foresee the scope of the conceptual revisions that will be necessary, nor the direction they will take. Thus a certain air of disorientation is only too understandable. Nonetheless, acquiring knowledge means exploring new hypotheses, new ways of visualising, without needing to obtain immediate confirmation. Starting from a set of premises to arrive at what can be proved on the basis of these premises has as its corollary that everything which cannot be derived from these premises is false. And yet we have to ask: does not the development of science in the course of the 20th century show that there is no such thing as knowledge underpinned by certain and unfalsifiable foundations? Why then should we limit our methods to the obligation of immediate proof? Surely it is clear to all that our knowledge increases when different perspectives begin to coexist, combining and integrating with one another, until a new truth content is produced? No discipline is self-sufficient, not even mathematics or physics: there are just so many components of a general system known to us as "nature". This is true for science in general, and all the more so for a science of consciousness, which obliges us to cast around for the most powerful theory, not the most elegant philosophy. All too often people insist that things should be "like this" and not "like that", whereas a researcher should always be open to different perspectives. Far from being a mark of eclecticism, such openness denotes humility, a sense of one's limits, the awareness of not possessing an exclusive or, worse still, "definitive" truth. What tends to prevail is the intransigent rhetoric of the determinists, on one hand, or of the seekers after the "heart of the matter" on the other. Consciousness can only be investigated from a plurality of viewpoints. And if, as must be apparent to all, our current knowledge does not allow us to grasp its inherent properties, then we should be looking for an explanation in which each particular discipline clarifies its own level of analysis, without trespassing into territories where it is neither conceptually nor empirically equipped to range.

For centuries humans have been interrogating time, the universe, consciousness. Each of these concepts stands at the edge of an abyss that is still unexplored. The closer we get to this abyss, the more reality seems to us ambiguous, elusive and fragmentary, and the more our convictions appear conjectural and provisional. Only the slenderest of bridges span the divide between the mystery of consciousness and the consciousness of mystery. It really would be begging the question to think we can avoid taking these bridges: they have to be crossed, and undoubtedly further bridges too. Not that we can hope to arrive at a goal that puts an end to the questions; we can, however, pursue the only goal possible, namely research.

CHAPTER
I

THE SPONTANEOUS ORDER OF CONSCIOUNESS

In this 21st century science is going to tackle the most baffling of all mysteries: consciousness. For thousands of years the question of consciousness has been bound up with mysticism and materialism, metaphysics and ontology, captivating and exhausting the mind of whoever has attempted to grasp its secrets, eliciting by turns feelings of exalted enthusiasm, beguiling confusion and bleak scepticism. But why should a phenomenon which is so familiar and yet so elusive be the mystery of mysteries? There are four main factors. In the first place the use of a single word – consciousness – is devoid of any empiric or conceptual demarcations; its multiple meanings have generated notable conceptual confusion, leading to uncertainty even in formulating problems and procedures and interpreting basic facts. Thus the same term* is used to designate such widely diverse phenomena as the condition of a patient in intensive care (in and out of consciousness), concern for the environment (ecological awareness), proper conduct (moral conscience), the activity of the ego (narrative consciousness) and a thousand other things besides. In the second place, the automatic identification of awareness – the state of openness to the world which informs our relational sphere – with consciousness. In the third place, the presence of qualitative states in conscious experience: the smell of a rose, the taste of a good wine, the sound of a piece of music and so on. And finally, the impossibility of agreeing on methodology among researchers who all take an interest in consciousness for various reasons but who have all too often proved unable to go beyond the boundaries of their respective disciplines while treating the 'physical' and 'mental' as distinct metaphysical territories.

For a long time consciousness was considered a biological property or

* Translator's note: the Italian "coscienza" can be rendered as "consciousness", but also as "awareness", "conscience".

function – comparable to the Krebs (TCA) cycle, circulation of the blood or photosynthesis of chlorophyl – which science would sooner or later succeed in clarifying, identifying the relative neuronal and synaptic activities and biochemical mechanisms. Even today there are scientists who are unwilling to recognise that consciousness originates in a neuron-based process that distinguishes the self from others; they are more at ease contemplating the complexity of the nervous system as such. Many factors favour the hypothesis that its success in evolutionary terms reflects the need of human beings to interact with their fellows, understand their intentions and thus enhance their possibilities of survival.

The terms of the question

Already Wilhelm Wundt observed that there is something tautological about the word consciousness. In common usage it indicates a broad spectrum of phenomena and psychical processes, even extending to the organization of our relational life. In its etymology, deriving from the Latin *conscientia* = *cum-scire* (knowing together), it evokes a relationship with another being or with the external world. Obviously, according to this definition any behaviour devoid of relational or communicative significance would reflect an absence of consciousness, although this inference does indeed appear questionable.

The term consciousness can have widely differing meanings the world over. In some cultures, above all in Africa, it is simply non-existent (Bleuler, 1961). In others, on the Indian subcontinent for example, it alludes to a fragment, as opposed to the Omniscient whole. In others still, notably in the Arab world, it indicates a knowledge of the interior universe, as invisible as it is essential. Then again one can recall all the meanings that have been laid down at the deepest levels of our cultural history: *syneidesis* (Holy Scriptures), *idea ideae* (Spinoza), *Bewußtsein* und *Gewissen* (which for some German authors possess a strong moral force). This overview could be extended indefinitely, but this is not the place for a detailed linguistic analysis. Not surprisingly, for many people this multiplicity of meanings has strengthened the conviction that consciousness is too difficult a concept to begin to investigate.

In reality, however, it is not impossible to identify a shared meaning, as long as one is careful to delimit the relative semantic field. Science differs from the other forms of knowledge for its ability to scrupulously define the objects of its enquiry. Certainly words have the task of indicating an object's function, but they also have to help us avoid the confusion that derives from semantic mistakes and from an ambiguous use of language. In common parlance, as in science, expressions and statements can be the source of ambiguities. Indeed, as Wittgenstein noted, ambiguities and misunderstandings are so much a part of our thought processes that very often we are not even aware of them. These deceptions would never surface if we failed to grasp the problems that underlie them. To the best of his or her ability a scientist, much more than a philosopher, has to throw light on the grey areas of language. Making an accurate definition of an object or a method of research has fundamental consequences for the import of a discovery. Of course no one can establish the limits of language, not least because they are inherent to language itself. Nonetheless, drawing a boundary between what can and cannot be said is perfectly within our capabilities.

Thus what are we to do about a term like consciousness that designates, at one and the same time, the highest manifestations of human ability and the normal state of everyday living? Should we use the term to indicate subjective consciousness, the oriented vigilance of a subject, or something else again? In medicine, for example, it can only be used in certain precise conditions: there must be an adequate state of wakefulness, an appropriate functioning of memory and attention, a good capability for discernment and decision-making, and correct temporal and spatial orientation. Another approach to consciousness takes account of the ability to have qualitative experiences (*qualia*), or again of a moral dimension. In everyday speech it is not uncommon to hear expressions like "I have a clear conscience", "the voice of conscience", "you've got a strong environmental conscience", "the character's conscience", "your conscience is troubling you", and so on. Similarly, in religious experience the term conscience alludes to a secret, intimate space, an inner recess where human beings find themselves alone before the transcendent. As in the context of qualitative experience, here too consciousness is an interior sphere that cannot be traced back to any roots. One further approach identifies consciousness with the mind (Gazzaniga, 1997), so that any intentional mental state is "conscious": a thought, a desire, a belief, a hope, a memory and so on. Strictly memory cannot automatically be attributed to consciousness, even though in the absence of consciousness memory would be fragmented in innumerable discrete experiences, without duration, brief instants of existence, as happens to patients affected by serious memory impairment. And so we could go on, but it is enough to recall a study by Miller (1950), still highly relevant even over half a century on, which listed no less than 17 definitions of consciousness in the scientific sphere alone.

The question remains: can a single word give expression to all these levels of meaning? The answer is clearly No. And yet today we are only able to say what consciousness cannot be: it cannot be a neurological process like vigilance; or a contingent reflex of the life of the mind, i.e. a subjective experience that is inaccessible to scientific appraisal; or again an abstraction of the life of the mind that can be assimilated to the Ego or to personality, merging into praxis and ethics and getting lost in the indistinct network of existential relations.

Milestones of a controversy

In tackling the problem of consciousness it is useful to form an overview, however incomplete, of the numerous theories that have succeeded one another in the history of this concept. Over the centuries fierce philosophical, religious and scientific disputes have hampered the formulation of a common standpoint, leading to a sedimentation of meanings that has made the term consciousness as polysemic as it is vague. At the same time, however, the idea we have of consciousness is very different from the one René Descartes came up with at the dawn of the modern age. On the basis of the distinction between *res cogitans* and *res extensa* (the fundamental principle of philosophical dualism) he argued that it is self-consciousness (*cogito*) which distinguishes us from animals. However fond humans may be of animals, they remain beings devoid of reason or awareness, incapable of pursuing truth, improving social living or contributing to the majestic edifice of civilization. During the Enlightenment many radically different theses were put forward by such determinists and fervent atheists as Julien Offray de La Mettrie (1709–1751), Claude-Adrien Helvétius (1715–1771) and Paul Henri Thiry d'Holbach (1723–1789), in which psychic phenomena were viewed as merely variants of the activities of the nervous system.

The debate really got under way at the beginning of the 19th century when the outstanding English neurologist John Hughlings Jackson (1835–1911) came out forcefully against the hypothesis of the existence of an entity called "consciousness". In his celebrated Croonian Lectures he took issue with William James's idea that consciousness is a function of the brain. He argued that "function" is a physiological term that is only applicable to biological events. The mere correspondence between psychic processes and cerebral events does not demonstrate that the former are a function of the brain. Nor, moreover, does the fact that the centroencephalic structures contribute to an effective relational existence automatically confer on them the role of "highest level". This role is the prerogative of the cortex, irrespective of the fact that, in order to manifest itself, psychic activity requires the structures to be perfectly functioning.

The clarity of expression and the strict correspondence between terms and concepts in the Croonian Lectures illustrate the care Jackson took over defining the relations between consciousness and subcortical structure. Although he was the first to speak of the 'highest level of integration' (a term which is still extensively in use, albeit in different contexts), he was careful to avoid expressions such as the "seat of consciousness". Long before modern neurological usage he claimed that the highest level (used, we should recall, in a conceptual not an anatomical sense) was represented by a neuronal system that is located in a number of places throughout the cortical associative areas; moreover, that the intermediate integration levels correspond to the sensitive or motor areas; and thirdly, that the lower levels are linked to the centres of reflex activity. One major implication of this model is that greater functional specialisation is matched by lesser plasticity, and vice versa, while this plasticity is very pronounced in the structures which are less functionally specialised, like the higher cortical structures.

Even though Jackson's original formulations were as clear as they were passionately argued, he has often been misinterpreted. He did not in fact attribute particular significance to localisation, as has been argued, and his functional mapping was by no means absolute. It is no coincidence that his conception based on the specialisation of certain neuronal areas remains perfectly valid today when the neurosciences have amply demonstrated the cerebral structures' remarkable and unpredictable capacity for compensation. Jackson was fond of saying that *there are no* independent functions represented at different levels, merely functions *that can be represented* at different levels. The famous German physiologist Emil Heinrich Du Bois-Reimond (1818–1896), an avowed materialist and strenuous opponent of the vitalism that characterised physiology in his day, maintained that the psychic processes stand outside the laws of cause and effect and thus cannot be considered on a par with cerebral activities. Proclaiming the motto *ignoramus et ignorabimus* [we do not know and will never know], he made no secret of his radical scepticism concerning the possibility of understanding the mysteries of nature and life, and first and foremost the relationship between the brain and consciousness. The Italian physiologist Luigi Luciani (1840–1919) was of much the same opinion, believing that psychic phenomena are not, as many maintained, the links in a chain of cause and effect running through natural processes. Just as Charles Sherrington (1857–1952) believed that the problem of the relationship between mind and brain will never be solved because thought is entirely immaterial, Luciani argued that it is highly unlikely that chemistry and physics will one day be able to make psychic phenomena intelligible.

The first person to postulate the existence of distinct levels in psychic activity – a subjective and an objective pole – was William Richard Gowers (1845–1915), an English neurologist and contemporary of Jackson, for whom the term "conscious" referred to the subjective sphere of psychic processes and the term "unconscious" to the exterior manifestations of these processes. This distinction has methodological implications, for we need both an introspective method to explore subjectivity, as in the practice of psychology and psychiatry, and another method based on objective observation, in the biological disciplines. Gowers had the farsightedness to grasp that a knowledge of psychic phenomena going beyond the merely superficial would inevitably imply integrating the two methods, even though the idea remains that consciousness is linked to the spontaneous mental activities: in practice, a patient is deprived of consciousness when these activities are absent and no sensorial stimulus can elicit them.

Stanley Cobb (1887–1968) made an interesting contribution to the emerging picture in claiming that consciousness is an attribute of the mind. Unlike the theory of various degrees of consciousness, Cobb envisaged a state of permanent variability, showing how models involving all/nothing or conscious/unconscious are fundamentally misleading. As the expression of the nervous system in action, consciousness involves awareness of the self and of the environment: it is a phenomenon that cannot be localised or indeed known, being inaccessible to our capacity for comprehension. Cobb's position was emblematic of how the difficulties posed by the issue of mind and brain not infrequently turn determinists into the most trenchant sceptics. In reality Jackson too had to admit that he had no explanation for the problem of consciousness, but this never made him a sceptic. On the contrary, he became increasingly convinced that there were precise natural laws governing its action. Showing a humility to match his scientific stature, he even expressed the fear that the knowledge he had accumulated might actually get in the way of the intuitive understanding required to solve this difficult problem. Jackson had grasped the role and the limits of the midbrain in the determination of consciousness, and as the 20th century advanced other eminent neurologists stressed its importance, coming to grant it the role of highest level. Julian de Ajuriaguerra (1911–1993) suggested, for example, that consciousness was underpinned by a basic dynamism associated with the operation of the Ascending Reticular Activating System (ARAS), which enables the individual to be an object in the sphere of phenomena and a subject in that of relationships. This viewpoint received its most authoritative endorsement from Wilder Penfield (1891–1976), the Canadian neurosurgeon who made his name by demonstrating, through the stimulation of small areas of cerebral nerve tissue, the existence of the motor homunculus, i.e. the representation of the various body systems on the motor and sensory cortex.

Penfield gave pride of place to the midbrain system in the organization of the higher functions. More specifically, he argued that the upper midbrain stem is the seat of consciousness. He cited three findings in support of this hypothesis: (a) lesions in those areas cause a loss of consciousness; whereas (b) ablation of even sizeable zones of the cerebral cortex do not affect consciousness; and (c) an epileptic fit generally has no influence on consciousness except when it affects the midbrain system. If these reasons should fail to persuade, Penfield added that isolation of one cortical motor area from the adjacent ones does not rule out the performance of a voluntary act. In this case, in fact, the impulse would traverse the only route still intact: the one connecting the motor centres to the midbrain system. This means that the highest level cannot be located in the frontal lobes. In his view the 'control room' of consciousness and will undoubtedly lay in the upper midbrain system.

Apparently the arguments Penfield used in support of his hypothesis – backed up by a considerable number of experimental findings – were sufficient to deter any attempt at confutation. Nonetheless the British neurologist Francis Walshe (1885–1973) set about doing just that in a celebrated article published in the journal *Brain* in 1957. After paying tribute to the sound work of researchers like Jackson and Sherrington – who made no secret of the fact that they had no solution to offer for the problem of the relationship between mind and brain, and hence consciousness – Walshe, in an evident challenge to Penfield, revived the concept introduced by the English physiologist William Benjamin Carpenter (1813–1885) that the thalamus/basal ganglia system is no more than an "automatic apparatus" which has little or no influence over the upper functions. Walshe saw little difference between the model put forward by Penfield and that of Carpenter. How would it be possible, he asked, for such a small, ancient area of the human brain to supervise the whole range of our physiological and psychological functions? In support of his standpoint Walshe referred to the thesis of the American neuropsychologist Karl Lashley (1890–1958) that there can be no nervous activity correlated with structures which are simpler than the underlying psychological activity. In other words, such an intense and sophisticated psychic activity cannot be supported by such limited neuronal areas. Indeed, the more extensive this activity, the greater the cortical areas involved have to be.

Now, while Carpenter could be justified on account of the limited knowledge of the hemispheric functions scientists possessed in the mid-19th century, there are no such attenuating considerations for Penfield. He was guilty of undervaluing the enormous number of discoveries concerning the functions of the nervous system that had been made in the course of a century and that had clarified, quite unequivocally, how cortical integration represented the climax of the development of the nervous system. And moreover, why should so much importance be attributed to areas that are as tiny as the intralaminar nuclei of the thalamus or the mesencephalic tegmentum? Questions must be asked about the importance given to the cortical stimulations carried out by Penfield on thousands of patients. An induced electrical stimulus cannot be likened to the natural influences the brain usually registers. In other words, the action of the cortex when stimulated electrically is by no means equivalent to the action of the cortex on the organism. Penfield, Walshe concluded, had actually set his sights on achieving one specific outcome: to overturn the natural order of the nervous hierarchies and assign to the midbrain the prime function performed by the cortex in the relational sphere.

Walshe's attempt to reassert the primacy of the cortex over the midbrain did not in fact detract from the immense value of Penfield's discoveries. The rather peevish and in many respects incomprehensible invective was anything but exemplary. Scientific debate is all about confutation, meaning the firm, measured demonstration of the untenability of a thesis or theory on the basis of circumstantial evidence or reasoning. Invective plays no part in this. Nonetheless, once the resentments have been allowed to discant, Walshe's *vis polemica* illustrates the keen, indeed passionate interest that the problem of consciousness has aroused in all those who dedicate a lifetime to probing its mysteries.

A major step forward in the investigation came with the work of the French psychiatrist Henry Ey (1900–1977), who perhaps more than anyone focused on the phenomenon of consciousness. He believed that consciousness is an activity whose expressions, degrees of reality and contents vary according to the circumstances of everyday life, with a hierarchy that can change quite freely. He argued that the whole spectrum of psychiatric illnesses can be seen as the consequence of a disorder of consciousness. In this conception, which is strongly influenced by Jackson's work, the de-structuring of consciousness can lead to a degeneration in the dynamic structure of the subjective experience. This process begins with a 'de-temporalisation' at various levels: first the projection into the future of the manic state and the withdrawal into the past of the depressive state; then the qualitative disorders of consciousness; and finally the disorientation in terms of time and space, seen in momentary fantasies, oneiric alterations combined with qualitative alterations, and formal disorders of the thought processes causing serious discriminative and cognitive alterations.

Ey brought to a close, we might say, the lengthy era of Victorian neurophysiology: no longer would it be possible to describe the nervous functions in terms of the old hierarchy of anatomical centres. The cerebral cortex becomes the locus for "optional exercises of the field of consciousness", while the midbrain is the neuronal infrastructure for the vertical plane of the sphere of consciousness. The activity of the cortex is based on vigilance, which represents its openness to the world. The distinction between the higher (cortical) levels and the lower (subcortical) levels has had its day. This does not mean that Ey failed to understand that the cortex is indispensable for the operations of the reflexive consciousness and the midbrain for the dynamism of the waking brain, and more besides. However, it is time to recognise that the terms and concepts in standard use have actually confined our reasoning in overly schematic frameworks.

A condition always at a far remove from equilibrium

The first person to come up with an evolutionary interpretation of consciousness was Herbert Spencer (1820–1903). The widely respected English biologist and philosopher maintained that consciousness arises out of the perception of the passage from one state of mind to another. It could never stem from an inert mentality. Moreover it differs from instinct only in degree and intensity. In fact while the manifestations of consciousness are extremely complex, those of the instinct are simple and stereotyped. The mind reveals itself by means of ascending evolutionary processes involving a progression from reflex to instinct, instinct to intelligence, and intelligence to reason. Later on in life Spencer modified his determinism, asserting that scientific knowledge is never definitive and that there will always be something that is unknowable beyond it.

The emergence of scientific psychology marked a rupture in the relations between philosophy and psychology. The opening of the first laboratories (in Leipzig in 1879 and then elsewhere) highlighted psychology's long felt need for autonomy. Boosted by its first experimental results, it was now determined to endow itself with an epistemological statute to match the other natural sciences. However, it could not get very far with the tools and methods available. Undoubtedly the introspective method made it possible to study feelings, desires and thought processes. But scientific methodology required them to be isolated and measured in terms of regularity and determination, and this was quite impossible. In fact Wundt was forced to admit that the higher processes cannot be investigated experimentally. Nonetheless he identified two dimensions of consciousness: the first was focused and distinct, the second general and confused. He used the term field of consciousness to designate the simultaneous awareness of contents in which activities like knowing, learning and so on merged into the stream of the immediate present as experiences that were happening on the spur of the moment.

William James attempted to transcend the opposition of spirit and nature. In *Does "Consciousness" Exist?* (1904) he wrote memorably that the only reality principle is the pulsing of experience. James did not go in pursuit of an abstract spirituality separate from nature. His aim was to free from rational time the instant that irradiates psychic life and disperses the mists of reality.

> What is true here of successive states must also be true of simultaneous characters. They also overlap each other with their being. My present field of consciousness is a centre surrounded by a fringe that shades insensibly into a more subconscious. I use three separate terms here to describe this fact; but I might as well use three hundred, for the fact is all shades and no boundaries. Which part of it properly is in my consciousness, which out? If I name what is out, it already has come in. The centre works in one way while the margins work in another, and presently overpower the centre and are central themselves. What we conceptually identify ourselves with and say we are thinking of at any time is the centre; but our full self is the whole field, with all those indefinitely radiating subconscious possibilities of increase that we can only feel without conceiving, and can hardly begin to analyze. (. . .) In principle, then, as I said, intellectualism's edge is broken; it can only approximate to reality, and its logic is inapplicable to our inner life, which spurns its vetoes and mocks at its impossibilities. Every bit of us at every moment is part and parcel of a wider self, it quivers along various radii like the wind-rose on a compass, and the actual in it is continuously one with possibles not yet in our present sight. (James, *The Works of William James II*: 760–762)

In *Essays in Radical Empiricism* (1912) James restricted the ego to the here and now, whereas in *The Principles of Psychology* (1890) the action of the ego was described in all its dynamic and temporal richness. James went into the attributes of character, individuality, creative force and orientation which, in merging together, gave rise to an identity that was open-ended and constituted over time. We can note, and we shall see in more detail later on, that James's exploration of consciousness bore significant affinities (as well as marked differences) with Husserl's *On the Phenomenology of the Consciousness of Internal Time* (1893–1917).

Some years previously the eminent French psychologist Théodule Armand Ribot (1839–1916) made an important contribution to the study of conscious processes. He maintained that consciousness is fundamentally the ability to reflect about oneself. In studies that have become classics, notably *Les maladies de la mémoire*, *Les maladies de la volonté* and *Les maladies de la personnalité*, Ribot illustrates the full extent of the difficulty of accounting for the complex reality of such categories as the ego, reason, will and memory. The ego, in particular, is not an entity but the sum of various mental events. Each of our conscious states is only a minimal part of our psychic life and is sustained by innumerable unconscious states. Compared with everything that remains submerged, what surfaces in consciousness is indeed only a minimal part. Ribot concludes with the admirable intuition that the unity of the ego is the effect of the temporary union of certain conscious states and innumerable unconscious physiological states which also operate and may indeed have more of an effect than the former.

Following in Ribot's footsteps, a brilliant pupil of his, Pierre Janet (1859–1947), put forward the hypothesis that consciousness is the effect of a combination of diverse events that give rise to a new phenomenon. He anticipated Freud in positing the existence of an unconscious psychic universe, arguing that psycho-pathological symptoms are the expression of dissociated unconscious material. Janet had grasped the thread that links the events of an individual's past life to the symptoms he or she presents. His contribution to the on-going debate with the elaboration of the concepts of dissociation and the subconscious gave an extraordinary impulse to Wundt's concept of field of consciousness, which Janet redefined as the set of phenomena that go to make up personality. Moreover he argued that alterations of consciousness are caused by the restriction of the attentive functions operating at any one time in the individual consciousness. These restrictions are particularly evident in the psychoasthenic syndrome in which attention – above all when it is polarised in terms of organic sensations – plays a crucial role. In his analysis of personality disorders the French researcher showed how the conflict between 'higher level' phenomena is manifested at a 'lower level'. At the same time, however, he warned that the term psychoasthenia must only be used in the clinical context: even then he was convinced that too much was being made of the unconscious. One and the same phenomenon cannot be used to explain both a condition and its cure. Improper use detracts from the creativity of consciousness, wrongly attributing it to the unconscious; this has the effect of causing the personality as a whole to regress to lower levels, even when it manifests itself in the highest expressions of artistic creation.

THE STRUCTURE OF CONSCIOUNESS

Methodological conundrums

Every day millions of people the world over enter and exit the state of consciousness. It is indeed striking that the knowledge and experience that has been accumulated in the sphere of anaesthetics has contributed so little to the on-going scientific and philosophical debate. Research in this field would help not only to bring this topic out of the operating theatre but also, and above all, to endow the *science of consciousness* with rather less tenuous foundations. For too long now debate has tended to focus on rarefied (and often irrelevant) theoretical controversies; it is high time to set about defining a set of consensus-based empirical procedures.

In general, investigation of consciousness refers to three basic levels: the neuronal correlates, the underlying causes of this correlation, and the reproducibility of the hypotheses produced. Clearly the existence of specific causal levels can only be verified in a healthy individual: in a patient suffering from altered states of consciousness the required monitoring, difficult enough in itself, would be out of the question. Nonetheless, even in the presence of all the conditions favouring the verification of precise causal levels and the necessary correlations between structure and functions, it would soon become clear that the nerve areas involved in conscious processes are also involved in other mental functions – both conscious and unconscious – like perception, attention, memory and so on.

So what are the optimal experimental conditions for a neurobiological study of consciousness? And how are we to adequately describe its contents if they can only be verbalised in the third person? There are behaviours, gestures and movements associated with neural activities that can be represented using electrophysiology or cerebral imaging. Several years ago Frith (2002) distinguished three levels of neuronal activity, associated with conscious representation, sensory stimuli and behaviour.

In the study of consciousness more than in other fields, theory has to go hand in hand with experimental research. Even if the formulation of accurate experimental models is always the first step, we can only gain a true understanding of the fundamental processes if we are familiar with the elementary neural levels. In recent decades studies of cerebral activation (using fMR, PET, MEG, event-related potentials) have made an extraordinary contribution. These techniques make it possible to explore cerebral reactions prior to and following a stimulus such as the presentation of ambiguous visual prompts, transition from a general anaesthesia to consciousness, passage from the vegetative to a minimally conscious state, and so on. For example, the renewal of the thalamo-cortical activity in a patient who was first 'vegetative' and then 'minimally conscious' confirms on one hand the importance of such connections in the processes of consciousness, and on the other that this cannot be circumscribed to one specific region of the brain.

Studies on the passage from oblivion to consciousness carried out in the sphere of anaesthetics with the help of cerebral imaging are making important contributions to our knowledge of conscious processes. In particular some very recent research work has shown how coming round after anaesthesia – with full recovery of a clear, oriented consciousness – is often preceded by a phase of considerable turbulence. Apart from all the questions that remain open, the demonstration of the co-implication of cortical and subcortical areas in the emergence of consciousness is an important step forward. Experiments conducted on twenty young volunteers coming round from a general anaesthetic by a research team led by Harry Scheinin (2012) have shown how the recovery of consciousness is correlated to the activation of profound cerebral structures rather than to the cerebral cortex. In other words, the state of consciousness is preceded by an intensification of the metabolic activities of the midbrain archipelago comprising the thalamo, limbic system and the lower frontoparietal cortical areas. The emergence of progressive levels of consciousness, monitored according to the response to vocal commands, right up to the highest level of consciousness of the self and the world, begins from these neural territories.

It is indeed extremely interesting that the activity of profound cerebral structures can also be elicited by anaesthesia. This suggests that there is a common autonomous mechanism of arousal. More generally the study of the effects of anaesthetic drugs and their ability to modulate consciousness opens up new scenarios for research. The suspension of the relational sphere and the passing into a state of oblivion on one hand, and the recovery of consciousness as the pharmaco-dynamic effect wears off on the other, constitute phenomena of extraordinary importance for a science of consciousness.

The passing of phrenology

Half way through last century Moruzzi and Magoun (1949) informed the scientific community of the existence of a system – comprising the reticular formation, thalamus and thalamo-cortical system of bi-directional projection – which governs the activities of wakefulness and vigilance: the Ascending Reticular Activating System (ARAS). In particular the two neuroscientists observed that stimulation of these areas causes a sleeping animal to awaken, and a state of alarm in an animal that is already awake. There are essentially two pathways for these influences: one extra-thalamic, responsible for the reactions of reawakening; and the other thalamic, which modulates the level of vigilance, orienting it in one direction rather than another. This second route appears to be more closely correlated than the first with attention which, as we can recall, is a selective phenomenon in relation to the higher levels of integrated nervous systems. It is vigilance that ensures the efficiency of attention and, more generally, the functioning of the entire psychic apparatus. In fact, in a non-vigilant subject not only attention but also other faculties such as memory, decision-making and motivation remain in a virtual state. Thus if reflex represents the lowest level of motor integration, vigilance represents the fundamental level of the higher integration which has the ARAS as its basic structure.

It is worth reiterating that the centrality of the ARAS in the organization of the central nervous system does not correspond to a hierarchical superiority with respect to the cerebral hemispheres: given their high specialisation and greater selectivity, they do their work at a higher functional level. Moreover, for specific anatomical and physiological reasons, systems with a specific projection (olfactory, gustatory, visual, auditory, somatosensory) have functions which are quite different to those of a system with general projection.

The former are made up of a peripheric receptor, afferent pathways and relay nuclei for these pathways which access a small portion of the cortex; and the latter of cellular aggregates distributed throughout the brain stem whose stimulation has a widespread influence on the electrical cerebral activity. The ARAS is not limited to the brain stem: it projects upwards towards the cerebral hemispheres and downwards towards the spinal cord. As Mauro Mancia (1994) pointed out, its functions are much more complex than simple cortical desynchronization, even though this is essential in the state of alertness and attention. Its thalamo-cortical projections, which are a-specific with a high oscillatory frequency, are fundamental for some essential functions of consciousness.

Studies of cerebral activation have shown that in patients in a vegetative state (i.e. wakefulness without content) the connectivity between areas that are normally connected is lost: in particular between the primary cortical areas and the associative multimodal areas (prefrontal, premotory and parieto-temporal, cortex of the posterior and precuneo cingolate gyrus); or between these areas and the thalami. This evidence taken together suggests that the vegetative state is a sort of disconnection syndrome in which an isolated neuronal activity is associated with a reduction of the cerebral metabolism (Midorikawa, Kawamura and Takaya, 2006). Conversely, in patients in a minimally conscious state the connectivity between primary areas, associative cortexes and thalami is maintained, so that the anatomo-functional apparatus required for conscious activity is intact. These studies of cerebral activation are opening up new scenarios. Recent research has shown how, in a subgroup of clinically vegetative patients, cortical activities of information analysis persist in such a way as to make the existence of levels of minimal consciousness plausible (Kotchoubey, 2007). On the contrary, the verbalisation of words – which automatically excludes a diagnosis of vegetative state – could represent a complex or automatism generated by little 'archipelagoes' of neuronal activity without consciousness (Laureys, Owen and Schiff, 2004). This however brings us back to a crucial question: how small do these little archipelagoes have to be for them to be non-thinking?

A long-standing controversy

Over the last thirty years the philosophical debate on consciousness has involved the distinction between an easy problem (i.e. how the brain and psychic organization generate consciousness), and a hard problem (i.e. the relation between the neurobiological processes and the quality of subjective experience) (Chalmers, 1996). A significant contribution has come even from those who, without making any concessions to dualism or forms of scepticism, have assigned a crucial role to subjective experience - thus denying the possibility of its naturalisation. The proponents of this thesis believe that the limits of our mind prevent us from penetrating the secrets of consciousness and grasping the qualitative elements of the phenomena. Even if we know that it is the brain which handles sentiments and the subjective quality of our thoughts, we shall never be able to clarify the enigma of subjectivity (McGinn, 1991).

Then again there are scientists who, making the link between cognition and intentional states, have placed experience and cognition on the same level, favouring a functional approach (Jackendoff, 1987; Baars, 1988; Dennett, 1991). In particular, they identify mental events and states (beliefs, wishes, desires and so on) as *functions* rather than specific neural *processes*. It is simply functional relations that hold together mental states, sensory inputs and behavioural outputs. For the adepts of computational functionalism (which has seen the development of the strong Artificial Intelligence programme) the mind resembles a computer programme. Functionalists argue that thought manipulates symbols inserted in a functional network which has much in common with computer processing. In such a perspective it seems quite plausible that experience derives from the combination of single (cognitive) modular units which are then inscribed in a variable theoretical framework, linked in turn to the emerging unit. Even though this hypothesis is ingenious and has had considerable success, it is profoundly ambiguous, for while on one hand it remains solidly grounded in the materialist model, on the other it recognises the reality of experience and mental activity because in order to validate a theory there must always be a third person.

For a long time authoriative cognitivists such as Fodor (1983) insisted that mental phenomena are to be considered only in quantitative terms and not in qualitative or subjective terms. In other words the mind functions by means of vertical structures (modules) which mediate between the output of the sensory-perceptive organs and the central systems responsible for more complex elaborations. Rather than exchanging information with the central structures or other modules, these genetically determined modules follow predetermined and unmodifiable calculation strategies. It has to be added that, although he never repudiated this theoretical framework, in a later phase of his research Fodor (2001) recognised that his theory was not able to clarify the more distinctive features and properties of the human mind adequately.

Conversely, for Baars (1997) the brain can be represented as a multitude of scattered microprocessors competing for access to a global workspace in order to filter, exchange and file information. Here distinct contents emerge from competitive and cooperative dynamics between neural groups that are transmitted and then brought into consciousness. The unitary character of such an experience is guaranteed by diffusion mechanisms rather than by the content transmitted. According to Baars, this model helps to distinguish the level of the specialised processors (unconscious) from that of the workspace (conscious), and above all to clarify the intentional filter which raises the integration and voluntary control of the attentive and ideo-motor spheres to the highest level. In other words the global workspace constitutes a sort of stable context-purpose, starting from which consciousness brings order to the multiple sources of knowledge and the innumerable interactions. While undoubtedly fascinating, Baars's model leaves several major questions unanswered. For example, what are the hierarchies of neuronal selection, and the dynamics of neuronal activity?

If the debate among cognitivists ran into major theoretical issues, neurobiologists were also facing serious problems. First of all they had to decide what were the ideal experimental conditions for highlighting the neuronal correlates of conscious experience. As we have seen, even the most radical materialists were obliged to admit that the only way of accessing qualitative experiences was through verbal report. The gap between the subjective account and the conscious experience is still very large. Language is the only, tenuous bridge between our thoughts and those of other people.

It was undoubtedly the work of Francis Crick, the biologist who with James D. Watson discovered the double helix structure of DNA, which revealed to the general public the full scientific scope of the problem of consciousness. In the mid-70s Crick decided to abandon his work in molecular biology and devote himself entirely to what he saw as the greatest enigma of them all: consciousness. He was convinced that the solution to this problem would come from experimental study of the electrochemical exchanges of neurons and the identification of the neural correlates of consciousness, i.e. the cerebral processes that are synchronised with the states and contents of consciousness. Starting from findings made by other neurobiologists concerning the electric oscillations in an interval of 35–45 Hz in a cat's neurons, Crick put forward the hypothesis that consciousness originates from the unification of the oscillatory frequency of a number of neural groups. The synchronisation of the discharges was supposed to consign the psychic content to the working memory (Crick, 1994), while consciousness is manifested in an intermediate zone of representations, distributed between a lower sensory level and a higher level of thought processes. In order to bridge this gap Crick suggested that beneath the conscious level a homunculus perceives the world through the senses, formulating, planning and performing the voluntary actions. As a matter of fact, at a later stage of his research Crick himself went back on this hypothesis. On the basis of experimental evidence relating to visual patterns in primates, he suggested that the phenomenon of (visual) consciousness depends on the neurons in layers V and VI of the cerebral cortex, with the mediation of oscillating thalamo-cortical properties. This type of consciousness is sustained by electrochemical activity in the visual areas, which projects nerve bundles directly onto the prefrontal areas.

Edelman (1989) argued that one has to distinguish between primary consciousness (a multimodal structure which combines various sources of information) and a superior consciousness which develops in parallel with language acquisition. The superior consciousness is the expression of a conscious self which organizes past and future and recalls and narrates its experiences, emancipating the organism from subservience to the here and now. While primary consciousness connects memory to current perception, superior consciousness operates a synthesis between the memory of special values and categories distributed in the temporal, frontal and parietal areas. Consciousness is seen as originating precisely in the dimensional and categorial interaction between the non-self (which interacts with the world through current experience and behaviour) and the self (which by virtue of social interactions acquires a semantic and a 'syntactic memory' for concepts). Learning takes place by means of the development of memories of the former system, for which the perceptive categories take on an extraordinary value.

Clearly Edelman's model implies the presence of an external observer who, by means of a symbolic alphabet, codifies and decodifies messages. The complexity of this system varies with variations in the functional organization: it is relatively low when the connections show a statistic distribution, and at a maximum when linked to specific neuronal groups. The higher the reciprocal information between each sub-set and the rest of the system, the greater the complexity. The core of conscious experience is constituted by a scattered neuronal aggregate which brings about integrations with a duration of about a hundred milliseconds. According to Edelman the integrative activities required by higher consciousness occur on the boundary between the thalamo-cortical system and the other cerebral areas. This autonomous dynamic nucleus – which cannot be identified either in the brain as a whole nor in specific cerebral areas, nor yet in any one sub-set of neurons – is both unified and differentiated: in other words it gives rise to correlations at a distance between different regions of the brain that can vary from one moment to the next, within one individual and between one individual and another.

Although unquestionably intriguing, Edelman's model does not take into account some fundamental problems. For example, if consciousness mobilises multiple cerebral territories (the reticular formation, thalamic system and so on) characterised by spontaneous relations, how can dynamics which are so different and far apart, "de-territorialised" as it were, give rise to the most extraordinary of natural phenomena? Jean-Pierre Changeux (1998) has argued on more than one occasion that at the origin of consciousness there is a globally integrated dynamic recruitment of representations characterised by both unity and diversity, variability and competition in a restricted neuronal architectonic space. This recruitment has to be extended to feature the coordinated operation of a set of neurons (relatively autonomous with respect to one another) that engenders such phenomena as vision, semantics and motor skills.

Such an anatomico-functional hypothesis attributes considerable importance to neurons with long axons which are particularly abundant in the cortical layers I, II and III, and present in large numbers in the prefrontal, dorsolateral and inferoparietal cortex (Changeux, 1998). In this model the frontal lobes are given a crucial role in conscious experience, simulating multimodal cognitive tasks. Using the Stroop test (based on an incongruence between the sense of a word and the colour of the ink in which it is written) researchers have shown that whatever the colour in which a word is presented, its meaning is enunciated in a relatively automatic fashion (Dehaene, Kerszberg and Changeux, 1998). This indicates that the neurons of the workspace are used, by trial and error, to control the elaboration of information by the processors from top to bottom, although they work from bottom to top. If computer simulation of the model can clarify the dynamics of selection of a global representation, it will also enable prediction of the dynamics of cerebral visualisation during the task performance. We shall come back to the assets and limits of the models referred to above.

Attention and the Pillars of Hercules

For all the formidable progress made in numerous fields by cognitive neurosciences, we are still in the dark about very many aspects of attention. One thing that is now beyond doubt is the multiplicity of processes that underlie it, for attention is involved in numerous other fundamental cognitive processes – perception, motor action, memory – and any attempt to isolate it in order to study its constant features is bound to prove sterile.

For over a century and a half attention was a crucial topic in neurophysiology and psychology. In the early days of scientific psychology it was viewed as an autonomous function that could be isolated from the rest of psychic activity. However, this idea soon came to be seen as inadequate. At the beginning of the 20th century researchers became convinced that attention underpinned a general energetic condition involving the whole of the personality. Within a few years the emergence of the Gestalt and Behaviourism paradigms caused these studies to be overshadowed, and it was not until the second half of last century that they regained their importance.

For a long time the debate was influenced by the hypothesis that attention constitutes a level of consciousness varying widely in extension and clarity, and only functioning in relation to its variations: from sleep to wakefulness, from somnolent to crepuscular, from confusion to hyperlucidity, from oneiric to oneiroid states, and so on. Subsequently other approaches of considerable theoretical importance linked attention to emotion, affectivity and psychic energy or social determinants. Yet what do we really know about attention, the sphere of our life which orients mental activity towards objects, actions and objectives, maintaining itself at a certain level of tension for variable periods of time? How and to what extent is attention related to consciousness? Why does only a minimal part of the information from the external world reach the brain even though the physical inputs strike our senses with the same intensity? And why is it that, although they enter our field of consciousness, most of these inputs do not surface in our awareness? It is well known that in the selection of stimuli, attention is strongly influenced by individual expectations. 'Anticipations' 'decide' which objects and events appear in our awareness, and which are destined never to appear. The law of interest regulates a large part of the selection of the objects and topics on which our attention is focused.

Now, if it is true that we pay attention to what touches our sentiments and emotions, it is also true that this attention – whether it is spontaneous, intentional or direct – is highly selective. The distinction made by James concerning the various aspects of attention, admirably taken up and systematised by Bruno Callieri (1980) in the spectrum of expectation, observation and reflection, is still extremely useful. *Expectant attention* prepares for action and is always conditioned by the expected events. It contemplates both modes of conduct or reflex activities in the short or long term in animal existence and intentional behaviours sustained by generic instinctive drives. There are animals, for example, which appear to manifest enormous patience in contexts that are highly specialised. One can think of the biological/instinctual expectations of birds and rodents which wisely conserve their food, of the leopard who delays action until the gazelle comes up close, of the spider who lurks in wait for its prey. Then one can think of all the situations of human consciousness in which attention appears to be an instinctual spur susceptible of modulation within certain limits: the hunter crouching in the hide, the fisherman waiting for the fish to bite, the marksman ready to fire at his target, the athlete in the starting blocks. This attentive modality has a duration which cannot be specified even though it cannot be prolonged *ad infinitum*: from split seconds to quite lengthy intervals. Whatever the scope, a state of intense vigilance, alertness and tension is in action. *Observant attention* indicates a distance between the subject and the surrounding scenario, which the subject registers in detail but with different degrees. Here, where interest and motivations play a decisive role, attention deploys its agents to the full, whether modal (perplexity, hesitation, tiredness, somnolence) or maintenance (as when driving a car on an empty road). Lastly *reflecting attention* is exercised on an interior object on which mental activity is fully focused. In the reflection, attention is expressed through knowledge of the interior universe. Such turning in on oneself implies a keen attention, as in pure abstraction, meditation and contemplation.

Are there physiological indicators of attention? There undoubtedly are. We can name the orientation response to a new stimulus: signs such as the dilation of the pupils, peripheric vasoconstriction, cerebral vasodilatation, arrest of the alpha rhythm in the EEG, and the substitution of the irregular beta rhythm. This state of psycho-physiological activation, known as arousal, varies across a continuum (from sleep to psychomotor excitation) and is decisive for the efficiency of a subject's performances. At low levels of activation the subject can be distracted, while very high levels cause a reduction of efficiency on account of the diminishing of attentive levels.

Initially the theory of levels of activation was studied by psychologists, and subsequently by neurophysiologists, who investigated its relations with the ARAS and influence on cortical activity. In fact the concepts of attention and level of activation are correlated but distinct. Activation is a state of the organism which occupies a continuum, while attention is a selective function correlated with the levels of activation. The degree of attention depends on the level of activation of the organism, which in turn is modulated by the peripheric inputs and by its internal conditions. Intense inputs solicit the attention to select the significant biological or psychological information. Psychic energy can be deviated to change the focus of attention, as when an unexpected object enters the senso-perceptive field.

The object of attention can only be investigated in an efficient nervous system. The central hub is always the cortex, even when the sensory inputs appear to take pathways far removed from the field of attention. The attention is sharply stimulated not only by the meaning and intrinsic value of the object but also by the variations and freshness of its perception. In the absence of alterations attention fades away, to the benefit of the imagination. It is a universal truism that novelty captures the attention while the reiteration of a stimulus is habit forming and can end by inhibiting attention. On the contrary, attention can be activated by prompts or thoughts which have an emotional or affective charge, confirming the role of the cortex in this process.

The most recent neurobiological research has revealed the extreme complexity of the phenomenon of attention. Experiments have been conducted concerning various aspects of the influence of individual factors on the speed of reaction and how reaction times differ when confronted by two synchronised stimuli coming from different sensory channels: duration and sustainability, intensity and degree, concentration and focalisation, or activation and "arousal" (Boring, 1970). It is common knowledge that attention makes mental states clearer, sharper, more aware. In this respect the relationship between attention and degrees of consciousness appears very close indeed. Jaspers (1913) identified the coexistence of similar elements: the magnetism of an object or topic; the clarity of the contents, with reflections which can be foreseen but can also be quite unpredictable and mysterious; the influence of cognitive, affective and motivational elements on these processes. Now, if the latter elements can, within certain limits, be objectivised, the impact of an object can only be registered by an introspective appraisal, while the clarity of the contents requires a critical awareness.

In general, while there can be no doubt that attention makes the psychic processes more efficient, it is not unusual for their acceleration (or intensification) to weaken attention to the activities that are not in focus. More accurate analysis is called for of the relationships both between spontaneous attention and immediate interest, and between voluntary attention and interests that are distributed over time. Freud maintained that attention is the expression of a series of dynamic mechanisms which act between perception and desire (1886–95). According to this approach it is the difference in tension between these two attributes which gives rise to thought and attention.

This schematic overview would be even more partial if one were to ignore the natural, cultural and social foundations of attention. For it is thanks to attention that memory can be considered a system in continuous evolution rather than an archive of static images. Remembering also has a sense of movement. Each new experience represents the possibility of preserving the traces of our past life, safeguarding our personal historical and cultural "novel" from oblivion. This is all the more true if we bear in mind that attention always means attention to something, pure "intentionality". Attention, that is to say, "intentionalizes" an object, combining with it in an immediate perception. It is precisely the nature of attention which shows how the life of the mind is not an undifferentiated entity but a set of relations in continuous perpetuation. It is attention that impels me towards objects, introducing me to the world of things, broadening my perception and accompanying me to the verge of consciousness.

Ex pluribus unum

The scientific and philosophical debate concerning consciousness has long been dominated by the dogma of the unity of consciousness. However, the idea that the human brain generates a single stable consciousness that remains permanent through time does not seem to correspond to the multiple and intentional nature of its contents. This internal plurality requires a discussion both of the mechanisms that unify the diverse contents and of the biomolecular mechanisms underlying the conscious experience. In general a plural model of consciousness is based on two fundamental elements: a process distributed through the cortex and subcortex, which sparks the activation of the contents; and the elaboration and representation of the contents, which are then brought into consciousness.

But what is the nature of the relationship between neurobiological infrastructures and consciousness? Is it plausible that the extensive contents of experience, instead of joining the central system moment by moment (or else being integrated in one global operation) contribute to the conscious experience and only subsequently reach the brain? Herein lies the difference between a monolithic and a plural conception of consciousness. In fact it is one thing to maintain that everything depends on the brain's elaboration of the information and contents acquired, so that they are routed, represented and finally brought to consciousness; and quite another to say that consciousness is the effect of a set of phenomena generated by precise cerebral dynamics. If the first model has the features of a hierarchic, pyramidal process, the second appears to be the evolutionary outcome of the integration of visual, auditory, tactile, proprioceptive and other experiences (Ramachandran, 2004).

For a long time now studies of the consequences of lesions to the brain and the ablation of some of its structures have shown how it is possible to lose the ability to register movement while conserving the other aspects of a visual experience intact; or, on the contrary, to lose the sensations of colours and conserve the movement and visual experience (Zeki and Bartels, 1998a). If on one hand these deficits of quality and phenomena help to clarify the degree and genre of the brain's functional specialisation, on the other they cast light on the way it works on a large scale, involving modalities and domains which reflect clear-cut and sizeable anatomic divisions: primary visual elaboration in the occipital cortex, auditory elaboration in the temporal cortex, projectual and memorial elaboration in the frontal cortex. The multiplicity of these levels also clarifies the plural nature of consciousness, in which the functional distinctions are reflected in limited anatomical *divisioni* and *loci* (for example, visual motion in area V5 or colour elaboration in area V4). Semir Zeki has proved the existence of a multiple asynchronous system of micro-consciousnesses starting from the simultaneous presence of the diverse events of a visual scene, perceived at asymmetrical time intervals (Zeki and Bartels, 1998b). For empirical reasons a plural model of consciousness seems a credible alternative to the unitary-undifferentiated model which reveals, as we shall see, its theoretical and empirical fragility above all when it comes to explaining the self.

Here however we come up against one major objection: if consciousness is plural, why do we have the sensation of being a single whole? How can this unconscious plurality be at the origin of the self? Providing an answer to this question means first of all clarifying what is meant by 'being a single whole', a problem that goes beyond this book. Without venturing into this territory, one can state that the self emerges when the individual dimensions of an experience are sufficiently representative, coherent and compact (Winson, 1986). In normal circumstances we experience a world of objects which are ordered in space and organized in terms of regularity and contents, within significant spatio-temporal schemes. More exactly there are extramodal contents (e.g. colour and form) and intramodal contents (e.g. proprioceptions), also at the level of representations intended for the self. Obviously the expression 'representative cohesion' does not refer to an invariable characteristic of the conscious experience but to the outcome of a laborious process of integration of the nervous system. The appearance of the self is in fact in relation to the mechanism that underlies and elaborates the plurality of the local contents generated by conscious experience. This could be the mechanism at the basis of the unification of the multiple levels of representation of the self on which our behaviour depends.

The constitution of the self could thus become the terrain for research and confrontation between phenomenology and neurobiology. This would allow us to rethink consciousness as a multiple unity rather than an undifferentiated entity. The sense of a consciousness that unifies is a question not of oneness but of representative cohesion. In turn, this cohesion could explain the genesis of the self from the brain's multiple representative activities, unified within a conscious field. The representation of the self as a multiple unity could have important consequences for a science of consciousness because it places the oneness within the multiplicity of the qualitative subjectivity, *providing a solution* for various theoretical and empirical problems. This conscious subjectivity would ultimately come to be seen as the echo of innumerable local neuronal dynamics and distributed cortico–subcortical phenomena. Of course, instantaneous unity and unification achieved through conscious sequences – as takes place in iconic memory (Kandel, 2006) – are quite distinct processes. For non-pathological forms of memory it is essential for the conscious sequence to have a precise order. For example, a complete phrase is determined by our ability to remember its beginning and, through the duration, to arrive at its conclusion, producing a coherent discourse (Squire and Kandel, 1999). In fact the instantaneous unit (in itself flow) inscribed in time (duration) is, as we shall see below, an essential element of consciousness.

III

AN INVISIBLE SOVEREIGNTY

Rationality is but a moment of answerability, a light that is like the glimmer of a lamp before the sun.

MICHAIL BAKHTIN

Ab exterioribus ad interiora, ab inferioribus ad superior.

ST. AUGUSTIN

The spark of a firefly, a minuscule beam of light, and all around inky darkness. More than a century ago William James gave this description of awareness, the singular psychic faculty – essential for our life, thoughts, self-image – which enables us to sense the profundity of things, the passage of time, the colours of experience. Awareness does not impose itself: it is present, spontaneous. It is the natural, rather than any particular, state of things. It was long believed to enable rationality to guide the choices, behaviour, reasoning of which we are so proud. Nowadays even the partisans of this thesis are not so sure. A growing volume of experimental evidence is showing how false it is to believe that our mind is provided with formal schemes of inference that enable us to draw valid conclusions irrespective of the contents of the premises. Over the last fifty years this problem has received new and surprising answers. It has been shown, for example, that many individuals unconsciously adopt rules which are quite different to those deriving from rationality. Indeed, it has transpired that rationality is not in the least a natural attribute or a faculty which is innate in our species, but a complex discipline that is attained (and maintained) only at certain psychological costs. Instead, what appears to be typical of our species is the ability to identify certain contradictions, analyse them, verify them and, if appropriate, reject them. It is precisely the exercise of rationality that leads us to recognise the limits of our mind and its haphazard capabilities. Again, the exercise of rationality causes us to rethink the role of the external limitations on human action, restoring their due importance to the internal limitations. The idea (actually rather disturbing) of a perfect rationality has had its day. Even the most ardent champions of an Olympian rationality appear to endorse the idea of a rationality that is conscious of its own incompleteness, ready to contemplate what cannot be rationalised. True, rationality has specific neuronal limitations, but it is also true that we are able to describe ourselves at a whole range of levels. It is the intertwining of these two aspects that gives rise to the most familiar and elusive of all our experiences: our selves. When we become aware of a perception, an idea or a thought we are always confronted by an enormous quantity of details and relationships which make the boundary between subject and object aleatory and ambiguous. It is impossible to formulate clear-cut descriptions of either subject or object. Each act we perform is reflected in itself. But this reflection does not tell us what we are or are not like. It merely tells us that it is possible to be as we are, and to act the way we act.

No light is cast at the foot of a lighthouse

We do not really know what awareness is, nor what it has to do with the tangible world. Even if we grant it a biological function, we do not know if it is merely the surface effect of a brain that evolved for other purposes. In practice, evolution has often produced mismatches: biology invented culture, but culture has not done much to improve human nature: one only has to think of the impossibility of eliminating aggressiveness, violence, warfare. In spite of the rapid and extensive corticalization of the human brain, its subcortical structures have remained more or less identical to those of our ancestors. For our good fortune, however, the extraordinary quantity of rational decisions which has led to the formidable edifice of human knowledge has been underwritten by a natural logic whose rules, for the most part unknown, have proved highly advantageous in evolutionary terms. In any case, even if the neurophysiological models appear insufficient to explain the function of awareness, it does have precise neuronal correlates which have enabled man and woman to achieve a sort of extended adaptivity.

It is surely reckless to maintain that awareness plays only a marginal role in human behaviour. This claim is the exact counterpart of the claims that attribute to awareness an excess of importance in our relational existence. The beam of awareness only spasmodically throws light on our actions, precisely as the Chinese proverb has it: "The foot of the lighthouse is in darkness." Certainly we produce the most logical explanations on the basis of experience. We distinguish what is conscious from what is not – an individual from a chair, or a person who is awake from another who is sleeping – but we overestimate the length of time in which we are really conscious of our actions. When you think about it, we are not even conscious of our non-awareness.

To give a schematic account, there are two types of awareness, one characterised by qualitative sensations, the other lacking them. Although perception makes us (qualitatively) aware of objects or facts in reality, this does not make it a particular experience. For example, we could be grappling with an abstract problem or a difficult algebraic equation and be conscious of it without any specific qualitative or emotional experience. In reality any number of the memories of our past life are devoid of affective resonance. But why are there experiences that are qualitative and others that are not? What is the essential nature of awareness? We have no idea. We only know that awareness enables us to understand our behaviour and match it to the most diverse situations. If we fail to grasp its multiple essence, we shall never succeed in understanding its true nature (Bencivenga, 2008).

So, awareness means experiencing multiplicity. But what is multiplicity? Certainly not the juxtaposition of inter-connected entities, as if in a static mosaic. Multiplicity is the simultaneous action of subject and object. Without simultaneity, awareness would be unthinkable. And yet, paradoxically, for much of our daytime lives we are absent to ourselves. One just has to think of the presence–absence we slip into while driving on a long car journey. Everything passes in front of our eyes – the most varied landscapes, houses, cars going the other way, curious looking clouds – without any awareness of our selves. We are all one with the car, the road ahead, the landscapes. We go on and on, mile after mile, absorbed in our thoughts. Only later on, and not without a certain surprise, do we realise we have driven for long stretches without even realising it. But what does "without realising it" mean? When it comes down to it, we have done nothing to break the highway code, nor have we risked going off the road. On the contrary, we may have taken difficult bends without the slightest hesitation. What was the level of our awareness? Did we take those bends consciously or unconconsciously? Were we perhaps conscious without realising it?

As a matter of fact, if facts and objects did not register with us, guiding our automatic responses, it would be impossible to live. Our ability to process data and information is drastically limited. And yet, merely registering is not enough. Just as it is not enough to pay all possible attention in order to have full awareness of things and of our selves. At most we can snatch fragments of awareness from the oblivion of non-awareness. Perhaps we could even become aware of not being aware. But we would go on ignoring the fact that we are in a blind spot, a zone which is inaccessible to thought alone. And consciousness? What role does consciousness play in all this? Clearly there are no lack of tasks: it intervenes in the actions in progress in order to expedite them; it extracts the relevant data from the available information so as to make the best decisions; it analyses the variables at stake in choices; it establishes new hierarchies of values, needs and aims in situations of conflict; it comes up with successful solutions to certain problems; it collects and elaborates new, different evaluations and draws the relevant consequences.

The multiplicity of levels of awareness is made possible by a spontaneous order in which the impulse towards unity alternates with another impulse towards multiplicity. It is a question not just of physical and chemical agents but of a stream of processes which have nothing to do with our models (not infrequently more complex than the reality they are seeking to explain) or with the terms we use to describe ourselves: the ego, self, subject, and so on. It is clear that this variable phenomenology revives the time-honoured question concerning the unity or multiplicity of consciousness and how it encompasses the whole set of images and emotions associated with the body. A monolithic vision identifies plurality as a regressive sign, minimising the influence of the unconscious universe on conscious life. Rather than standing in a dialectic relationship with each other, awareness and non-awareness have a relation of profound co-implication, even of identification. The core of awareness is haunted by shadows, fantastic refractions, sudden illuminations which give us the illusion that it is the ego that is making the decisions, when in actual fact it is a matter of elusive dynamics that are inaccessible to our reasoning.

Awareness re-emerges, each time, in the interludes of thought, in the self-effacing states of meditation, in the unexpected flashes of non-awareness. There is a spontaneous, unexpected, sudden non-awareness. As when, in the orderly progress of our lives, something we weren't expecting suddenly bursts upon us, changing the order of things. The stability we believed we had attained is transformed into the absence of stability; the ground is cut from under our feet; we find ourselves in free fall. Later on, thinking back to that instant from the security of a regained stability – as in a sort of "shipwreck with spectator" (Blumenberg, 1985) – we will say that in that moment we were felled as if struck by lightning. Then there are events which make us unaware in a different way. Disturbing, chaotic events and fantasies which produce strong inner emotions and make us experience a life in which we are caught up without being so conscious of the fact: life at its most physical, involving a rush of bodily sensations. Here it is not a question of awareness of the ego but something deeper and more indistinct which hovers in the zones between consciousness and unconsciousness. Among these illusory refractions of transparency and opacity, awareness constitutes itself as the ego in a continuously changing perspective. But we need to be careful. This is not the passive spectator ego of an imaginary Cartesian theatre but rather an ego that achieves the highest degree of openness to the world of values, norms, decisions, liberty. It is starting from here that thought turns to itself and to things in general, i.e. not from just any abstract point but from a precise here (and now), part of lived experience.

But is there one fixed point at which we turn in on ourselves? This can be reached only if we turn our backs on the things around us. Neglecting the eruption of unmediated life would mean remaining cut off from the universe of awareness. The here and now of unmediated life goes beyond the limits of the body. One only has to think of the extraordinary value of the exclamation "I am beside myself". Our presence always asserts itself between a *from where* (past) and a *towards where* (future). Being means being here and, at the same time, being there. I am here, in a space. But I am also there, where I can see or touch something. And it makes no difference whether or not I pay any attention to that something. Things are here for me, I have them to hand. It is not even necessary for them to be within range of my perception. They are here for me together with the other objects, whether real, familiar or unknown. This external space of the body does not exist anywhere, or rather, it is the here with respect to which there is a there. It is a space where things have a place, in which we take our place. An oriented space, full of routes that can be taken and obstacles that it is more or less feasible to avoid. In order to transform those objects into a clear vision, in sensory perception, one just has to pay attention. Perceiving is seizing. Leaving behind the bodily dimension renders the sense of this eruption perfectly. It allows us to supersede the prospects granted to us, making us acquire others even though we remain motionless. The existence of Monte Tabor did not deny Leopardi the endless spaces. Limits are not there only to be transcended but in order to make up for the body's finiteness. We are body, but also more than body. We perceive, but we also know we perceive. We live from cradle to grave, but we also know that we were born and will die.

The awareness of awareness

It is almost impossible to talk about consciousness without talking about the quality of our experience of the world. Over the last fifty years this aspect has been a real bone of contention, above all among philosophers. At the heart of the discussion there is the concept of *qualia*, adopted by philosophers of the mind to indicate those perceptive experiences characterised by the presence of colour, sound, taste or whatever. One question has been whether *qualia* only occur in emotional states and in feelings, or in other states of mind too such as thoughts, utterances, beliefs. No one can deny that our thoughts are often impregnated with them. When we let out an *Aaah!* of joy, exaltation, even ecstatic rapture at having a hypothesis confirmed, are we really able to separate our selves from the quality of that experience? It is frankly difficult to think of an experience without a subject. And even more difficult to think of a subjectivity without an experience. There always has to be someone "in the first person" to have the experience of something.

How then are we to conceive of *qualia*? In at least two senses: the first concerns the subjective nature of the bodily sensations and perceptions; the second concerns the unintentional properties of some mental events. In the philosophical milieu the discussion has involved above all the phenomenic features. Thus when asked "Do consciousness and the mind act intentionally?", philosophers including Michael Tye, Fred Dretske, Tim Crane and William G. Lycan all gave a clear answer, albeit with different emphases: a mental state, an activity or an inner disposition are always "intentionalized" towards an object. A desire is always the desire for something. A thought is always the thought of something. Consciousness is always consciousness of something. In short, whether it regards perception, imagination or thought, the relation between the ego and objects is always intentional. The path to *qualia* is a sophisticated process which ascends all the way to being aware of an awareness of sounds, colours and much else besides. If this were not the case it would be difficult to attribute qualities to our experiences. And anyway, we have to ask: is our mental life part of objects or of experiences? Because if it is a part of objects, it must have a non-relational meaning and the mind itself must be none other than a cold network of nodes which are functionally autonomous. But this clashes with the hot, relational way in which we represent our mind.

In an article that has become a classic, entitled *What does it mean to be a bat?*, Thomas Nagel argued that it is impossible to reduce consciousness to mere neurobiological activity, so that no attempt at naturalization will ever be able to tell us anything about the subjectivity of the human mind.

> Conscious experience is a widespread phenomenon. It occurs at many levels of animal life, though we cannot be sure of its presence in the simpler organisms, and it is very difficult to say in general what provides evidence of it. [. . .] But no matter how the form may vary, the fact that an organism has conscious experience at all means, basically, that there is something it is like to be that organism. There may be further implications about the form of the experience; there may even (though I doubt it) be implications about the behavior of the organism. But fundamentally an

organism has conscious mental states if and only if there is something that it is to be that organism—something it is like for the organism. We may call this the subjective character of experience. It is not captured by any of the familiar, recently devised reductive analyses of the mental, for all of them are logically compatible with its absence. It is not analyzable in terms of any explanatory system of functional states, or intentional states, since these could be ascribed to robots or automata that behaved like people though they experienced nothing. [. . .] I do not deny that conscious mental states and events cause behavior, nor that they may be given functional characterizations. I deny only that this kind of thing exhausts their analysis. Any reductionist program has to be based on an analysis of what is to be reduced. If the analysis leaves something out, the problem will be falsely posed. It is useless to base the defense of materialism on any analysis of mental phenomena that fails to deal explicitly with their subjective character. For there is no reason to suppose that a reduction which seems plausible when no attempt is made to account for consciousness can be extended to include consciousness. Without some idea, therefore, of what the subjective character of experience is, we cannot know what is required of physicalist theory. While an account of the physical basis of mind must explain many things, this appears to be the most difficult. It is impossible to exclude the phenomenological features of experience from a reduction in the same way that one excludes the phenomenal features of an ordinary substance from a physical or chemical reduction of it—namely, by explaining them as effects on the minds of human observers. If physicalism is to be defended, the phenomenological features must themselves be given a physical account. But when we examine their subjective character it seems that such a result is impossible. The reason is that every subjective phenomenon is essentially connected with a single point of view, and it seems inevitable that an objective, physical theory will abandon that point of view. (Nagel, 1974, pp. 436–437)

Essentially, Nagel asks: What do living beings endowed with sensory apparatuses as different as those of humans and bats share? Or more simply, what do we have in common with creatures that are different from us? We have to admit that there is still no theory or phenomenology concerning "us" and the relationship between us. In any case, only a bat is able to see a bat's world. Even if we knew every detail of its nervous system, we could never know what type of experience it has of the world. Having a consciousness, Nagel maintains, means feeling oneself to be that specific being: i.e. a subject. But in fact, if we think of the subjectivity of a bat, it is obvious that we will never know what it feels like to be an individual different from us. The question concerns every intentional sphere, but also states like pain – an experience on the boundary between first person (the patient's reports) and third person (the biomedical records) – or the condition of patients suffering from serious sensorial and perceptive impairment (altered states of consciousness, minimally conscious states, coma, vegetative state) about which we know practically nothing. How many times, in the cold aseptic environment of an intensive care unit, have doctors and carers wondered if the absence of consciousness has cancelled out all trace of subjectivity in the patient. It is clear that if we adopted the on/off model – i.e. if research continued to focus only on the poor functioning of vigilance – every subjective trace and all the contents of consciousness would be cancelled. But in this way we would only confirm the thesis that is implicit in the premise, without in any way understanding the significance of "being not conscious".

Saul Kripke has argued that pain is only a state of the mind, remaining entirely autonomous from its somatic correlates and different from any other bodily experience or cerebral process. According to the American philosopher, dualism is fallacious for many reasons. The very identity of mind and body is only plausible in a highly abstract *monde possible*, which in any case would differ from all the others even if only in a single detail. In the passage from one world to the other, entities like mind and body would prove to be too rigid. To avoid contingency and caducity, the mind ought to be identical to the cerebral states in every possible world. But this is false, on the one hand, and logically impossible on the other (Kripke, 1971).

In this debate, the position of Ned Block (1978) is very interesting. He takes issue with the functionalist theory which represents mental events as algorithms that can be carried out by any machine capable of performing the necessary sequences. According to the exponents of strong Artificial Intelligence, computers are in fact much more than a means for studying the mind: they are themselves a mind. If properly programmed, a computer could not only carry out cognitive tasks but would even be able to understand (other) cognitive states. Block dismisses this thesis as mere conjecture. Citing experiments involving mental exercises – referred to as inverted *qualia* and absent *qualia* – he shows how the functionalists are not even able to describe such essential experiences as the perception of colour and pain. By definition a mind has to have qualitative experiences (Block and Fodor, 1972). To identify a mental state with a machine requires breaking the mind down into functional sub-sets which are programmed and assigned to homunculi with minimal work capacity. But, Block asked, could a set of computational functions generate the extraordinary diversity of experiences of which the human mind is capable? Granted that the idea of these homunculi operating like our mind is plausible, at both the microscopic and macroscopic levels, we would find ourselves plunged into a perfect paradox.

What Mary didn't know

In a celebrated imaginary experiment, Frank Jackson (1986) describes the singular story of Mary, a scientist who from birth was kept sequestered in a black and white room. Her entire relationship with the external world was mediated by a black and white screen. Mary's formidable knowledge of the laws of physics, chemistry and biology enabled her to unlock all the secrets of seeing colours: wavelength, the reactions of the nervous system to external stimuli, the construction of mental images, the colour of objects. Moreover, Mary also had an excellent knowledge of the structure of the human mind. So Jackson asked himself: what would happen if Mary were allowed to see the universe of colours about which, at least in theory, she knows everything? Would she learn anything new? And what effect would the colour red, for example, have on her? If red was a physical fact, it could be classified, in common with all the other facts she already knew. But Mary was having her first experience of the effect of red, along with many other things in the world. Her excellent knowledge did not suffice to give here a clear idea of reality. Like any other qualitative experience, colours cannot be described only in physical terms. Jackson concluded that there are facts and forms of reality which are extraneous to the science of physics. Although all sorts of objections have been made to Jackson's case study – on the type of knowledge Mary acquired before and after her liberation, on the objects of this knowledge, and so on – it is undeniable that an experience, of whatever nature, always introduces us to something new. A materialistic interpretation of the *qualia* does not explain how we get to the heart of an experience. Of course, similar considerations to those regarding colours could be made for perceptive experiences, bodily sensations and many other phenomena. At this point we can reformulate our questions more precisely: how does the brain produce qualitative subjectivity? And what lies beyond the neurons?

CHAPTER
IV

THE INTEMPORALITY OF CONSCIOUNESS

> To look for the essence of life in space is like trying to look for the path of the ship in the water: it only exist as a memory of the flow of its uninterrupted movement in time.
> The places where we happen to be are ephemeral and fortuitious settings for our life in time, and to try to recapture them is impossible.
> MARCEL PROUST

In the course of evolution, biological life on our planet has activated two strategies for adapting to the passage of time. First of all it inscribed elements in the genetic code which could facilitate an adequate flexibility in the face of environmental changes (light, temperature, precipitations); in the second place it endowed the animal nervous system with structures which can guarantee the sensorial and motor activities triggered over time. Compared to the higher order of animals, consciousness has also enabled humans to develop the capacity for an inner representation of time which has had great benefits in terms of adaptation and reproduction. In fact, the consciousness of time took longer to form than the consciousness of space. Many centuries passed before time lost its metaphysical character and became a subject for research like other natural phenomena. Modern science became able to distinguish the time of everyday experience from time as envisaged in religion and philosophy. However, for no real reason, at least up until the beginning of the 20th century, psychiatrists, neurologists and psychologists in particular paid much more attention to the mental perception of space than of time. Because if it is true that the experience of time is different from the experience of space, it is nonetheless of the same essence. The sense of time and, more in general, temporal experience is a quality of consciousness and should be investigated as such.

The intuition of the instant

James argued that we can only know the phenomena of the mind in terms of evolution and adaptation. There are two routes: the first, introspective, through observation and analysis of one's own feelings, emotions and so on; the second, through study of the relationship between consciousness and the environment. Our thought is the expression of a permanent and changing relationship with the objects that are independent of it. James rejects the idea that sensations are the elementary data of consciousness and that they give rise, through ascending dynamics, to ever more complex and refined levels of consciousness. Even an elementary perception, he maintained, is the effect of a subtle abstraction. The stream of consciousness – a concept that was to have an extraordinary influence on the work of such writers as James Joyce, Virginia Woolf, and Henry James – describes transits of thought from one object to another. There are no interruptions in thought, or at least no more than there can be, as James expressed it with a fine metaphor, in the knots of a bamboo cane. No psychological analysis can grasp the deep workings of the mind. No description can completely render the breadth and profundity of an experience, and the words and images used about it are cloaked in an aura which makes the description much less distinct than appears at first sight. In each experience, James says poetically, resounds "the dying echo of whence it came to us, the dawning sense of whither it is to lead" (1890, p. 255). It is not only the continuity of conscious life that is involved but everything new that flows into it. At each instant innumerable processes are being superimposed on one another in our brain, giving us the sensation of duration. The most remote moments leave behind them a wake that anchors them to the present moment. In this deceptive present, fragments of memory, both recent and remote, blend with the present experience while the echo of moments that have just passed reverberates in other moments in time that are about to happen. In this way the meanders of time past are joined up with time present and time future.

How often have we tried to make time stand still! It's easier to seize a ghost by the tail. Where is this present? Even before we've been able to imagine it, it's gone for ever, without leaving a trace. We can only sense its presence, as part of life. We have no senses we can use to identify it. We know it exists, even if we shall never experience it directly.

> The relation of experience to time has not been profoundly studied. Its objects are given as being of the present, but the part of time referred to by the datum is a very different thing from the conterminous of the past and future which philosophy denotes by the name Present. The present to which the datum refers is really a part

of the past — a recent past — delusively given as being a time that intervenes between the past and the future. Let it be named the specious present, and let the past, that is given as being the past, be known as the obvious past. All the notes of a bar of a song seem to the listener to be contained in the present. All the changes of place of a meteor seem to the beholder to be contained in the present. At the instant of the termination of such series, no part of the time measured by them seems to be a past. Time, then, considered relatively to human apprehension, consists of four parts, viz., the obvious past, the specious present, the real present, and the future. Omitting the specious present, it consists of three . . . nonentities — the past, which does not exist, the future, which does not exist, and their conterminous, the present; the faculty from which it proceeds lies to us in the fiction of the specious present. (James, 1893, p. 609)

The present is an isthmus of land from which we look out on time. Duration is the name we give to the incessant flux of the past into the future and the future into the past. It does not mean feeling a before and an after; in fact we are not aware of the passages between the successive moments. We perceive the intervals and the limits as a single whole. The distinction between the beginning and the end is pure illusion. Even if we pay all possible attention, we cannot separate the elements of our perception.

And in any case, rather than mirroring the data of reality, consciousness is an "intelligent intelligence" projected onto the world, susceptible of both successes and failures. It is the actor of the projects and enterprises undertaken by experience. It invents concepts, perceives hidden relationships, recognises resemblances and much else besides, exercising an activity which, however, does not possess that "legislative power" which Kant attributed to the rational mind as opposed to experience. The idea of objective time, as an infinite and necessary continuum, is unfounded. Time cannot be reduced to the causal order of space. At the origin of the consciousness of time there is the intuition of duration.

Neuronal melodies

There is general consensus among neuroscientists today that our perception of time originates in the different pace at which we perceive changes over a specific interval, relying on minimum correlation thresholds between neural processes and cognitive events supported by wide-ranging integration with diffused synchrony. More accurate knowledge of these correlations could clarify both the nature of the local events and the process of global synchrony which lies at the heart of an experience.

There is still no agreement about the nature of the processes underlying the phenomena of succession and duration. For over 150 years it was believed that the extent of the interval between certain events was the real key to the cognition of time, and enquirers failed to grasp the difference between the succession of neuronal events and the order of this succession. The succession of acts of consciousness is not the consciousness of their succession. We need other models to explain why our states of consciousness are accompanied by the consciousness of their succession.

Acceptable hypotheses on the nature of the perception of succession and duration indicate the following orders of magnitude: beneath 100 milliseconds it is possible to distinguish the beginning and the end of an instantaneous event, while beyond 5 seconds the perception of the duration in memory appears to be halved (Fraisse, 1987). Francis Crick and Christopher Koch (1992) identified a mechanism of temporal unification of the neuronal activities as the basis of consciousness, believed to synchronise the impulses in oscillations averaging 40Hz. Rather than codifying additional information, these oscillations are supposed to bring together part of the existing information in a coherent perception. In reality, in a subsequent phase of his research Crick questioned the idea that these oscillations were sufficient to generate a conscious experience, referring to other explicative hypotheses and more complex models of connection.

Apart from the question of the specific frequency of the talamo-cortical oscillations, there no longer seems to be much doubt about the fact that at the origin of consciousness there is the simultaneous action of cortical–subcortical neuronal populations rather than a single cerebral area. As has been shown by various electroencephalographic studies, these are multiple neuronal circuits, activated by phenomena of parallel synchronization and inhibition: transitive and substantive states characterised, in the former case, by an instable, high energy neuronal activity, and in the latter, by a stable, low energy neuronal activity. This gives rise to a dynamic equilibrium in which each event (an abstract thought, a visual image or whatever) reflects the activation of a neuronal network, distributed and in parallel, which creates contents of consciousness (Le Van Quyen et al., 1997). Neuronal oscillations play a decisive role in this talamo-cortical communication. Experimental evidence shows how some physiological states (going to sleep, wakefulness, vigilance) and certain pathologies (depression, epilepsy, Parkinson's) are associated with different talamo-cortical rhythms, whose duration varies according to variation in the clinical populations. In paranoid schizophrenics, for example, they are more short-lived; in maniacal patients they manifest continuous changes in rhythm (Goodwin and Jamison, 1990), and so on.

In any discussion of consciousness metaphors come in very useful. Let us try for a moment to imagine the brain as a musical ensemble. Everyone knows that the success of a concert is linked to the synchronised performance of the musicians rendering a particular score. But how does a score become melody? A melody is much more than the notes that go to make it up. In fact it arises out of the mysterious coming together of frequencies, rhythms, accelerations – it does not come from merely combining them. The combination of the notes of the strings and the piano, the rhythms of the percussion instruments and more besides, provide an accurate simile for the oscillations of neurons, their harmonies and disharmonies. Now, while this model is certainly not adequate to explain the emergence of subjective consciousness, at least it stops us having to call on such metaphysical entities as the "central theatre", the homunculus or whatever. This is how subjectivity could arise from the organization of neurons, according to evolutions and variations which, as in a symphony, accompany the orchestra without ever being identified with it.

It does indeed appear highly promising to collocate the problem of consciousness in a temporal perspective. Time helps us to be more rigorous in our consideration of decisive experimental aspects such as the significance of the use of time scales based on milliseconds which render the unity of the conscious experience no more than an illusion. On these time scales immediacy, a category that is all too readily attributed to consciousness, disappears. There are in fact processes which are apparently insignificant on account of their infinitesimal duration which instead possess enormous scientific value. At least half a second has to elapse from its arrival at the cerebral cortex before any information can access consciousness. Now we can turn to the apparent tardiness of "conscious consciousness".

Retrospectives of time

To say that consciousness is slow-moving apparently runs counter to common sense. A large part of our actions and movements take place extremely fast. Besides, if consciousness were slow, how could our ancestors have implemented those rapid decisions, showing a remarkable degree of adaptability, which ensured our survival? In a series of brilliant experiments conducted between the late sixties and the end of the eighties using electrical stimulation of the premotory cortex in patients undergoing neurosurgery, Benjamin Libet demonstrated that although stimuli lasting less than about half a second trigger the expected neurophysiological reactions, they are not consciously perceived. In particular he observed that our brain seems to know that we intend to perform a certain action half a second in advance.

> If you tap your finger on a table, you experience the event as occurring in "real-time". That is, you subjectively feel the touch occurring at the same time that your finger makes contact with the table. But...the brain needs a relatively long period of appropriate activations, up to about half a second, to elicit awareness of the event. Your conscious experience or awareness of your finger touching the table thus appears only after the brain activities have become adequate to produce the awareness. (Libet, 2004, p. 32)

Thus consciousness is delayed with respect to one part of our brain, and the impression of having decided to perform an action is totally illusory. Libet put forward the hypothesis that consciousness arrives when the action is completed, whether in terms of the sensorial input or the motor output. The "readiness potential", an expression of the electrical activity in the brain that immediately precedes the performance of a complex motor act, sets in motion the codification of the programme of muscular–skeletal actions necessary for the action. In an ingenious experiment Libet demonstrated that if a movement is preceded by the decision to act by about 200 milliseconds, the readiness potential is preceded by about 550 milliseconds.

Over the years Libet's findings have met with significant objections. The first concerns the fact that subjective verbal reports do not tally with evidence concerning the action potentials of cortical activation which correspond to sensations and movements. It is difficult to identify free will with a mere veto on a motor act already in course without an empirical validation of a conscious process. The second objection queries the plausibility of the experimental task, involving a ballistic movement that is to some extent pre-programmed, having a veto as a congruous voluntary act.

Attention was focused once again on consciousness as the causal agent of events by Patrick Haggard in his work on reaction times (Haggard, Clark & Kalogeras, 2002). This research was based on the premise that the intention, programming and performance of a movement and the anticipation of its sensorial consequences are in a sequence made congruous by the brain activity. To verify this hypothesis the authors, like Libet, used a clockface and reports in which the subject communicated the instant at which a conscious experience began. Four phenomena were examined: (a) a voluntary act (the subject had to press a button registering the performance time); (b) an induced contraction (the subject had to register the starting time of an involuntary contraction provoked by transcranial magnetic stimulation); (c) an induced sensorial phenomenon (the subject had to register the time in which an auditory sensation took place, a sort of click produced by transcranial magnetic stimulation); and (d) a naturally induced sensorial phenomenon (the subject had to register the time in which a normal auditory sensation took place). In a second series of experiments, the same events were related to the subjective perception of the time interval that passed between the event itself and an audio stimulus administered 250 milliseconds later.

The overall results of these experiments showed how, in the case of voluntary actions, consciousness of the motor act was delayed, while consciousness of the related audio event was anticipated, making for a substantial bracketing of the two events. Whereas in the case of an induced contraction, there was an opposite effect to the delayed perception of the related audio event. In this process the single events are apparently integrated and unified into a coherent conscious experience (Haggard et al., 2002). These experiments demonstrate how, in temporal perception, our brain constructs parts of reality and how, for its part, consciousness supports the self as the actor (albeit often arbitrarily) of the events in an action or sensation.

Irrespective of their historical importance, the findings of Libet and Haggard (and many others too numerous to mention here) suggest that at the basis of consciousness there is a sort of synchronization between different regions of the brain, and that this temporalization is decisive in the processes of integrating the information received from the neurons. However, no one is able to say anything about how the passage from the neurons to consciousness takes place. This is why it is vitally important to seek new experimental proofs for the hypothesis that at the origin of "global objects" there is a causal implication of the local events and a minimum time required for the neuronal events related to a cognitive event to transpire. When viewed as the origin and structure of consciousness, time is the direct link joining up the various levels of neurobiological research and phenomenological reflection. This is why we now need a significantly different terminological and conceptual register.

The intemporal structures of consciousness

In *Time and Free Will: An Essay on the Immediate Data of Consciousness*, Bergson (1889) confronted the spatialized vision of duration held by the positive sciences with actual duration. Long before him the Eleatic philosophers, and subsequently Augustine, had attempted to throw light on the concept of the present, querying the notion of time as a succession of present moments. The term Bergson assigned to the experience of time – an experience with qualitative, dynamic, discontinuous and asymmetric features – is "duration". He maintained that the explanation of time given by physicists is totally erroneous. The symbolic time of mathematical equations does not correspond to real time. At best it is an abstraction, a mere succession of moments placed one beside another, like separate segments, identical one to the other and indifferent to content.

Our experience of time, on the other hand, is duration, change, flux, a continuous and uninterrupted stream. The key to the experience of time, he argued, lies in the immediate data of consciousness, in the flow of sensations and perceptions which succeed and merge into one another tirelessly. Time cannot be thought of as a string of pearls, with one event next to another. Human time is made up of phenomena that are so rapid that we do not perceive change. After all, if the analogy of the string of pearls were grounded in fact, nothing would exist beyond the present moment. As soon as it is over, a perception would vanish for ever. We would never acquire experience of anything. And even if there were some order in our ideas, we could not be aware of it. One idea would simply follow on from another, and that's all. Each state of consciousness, as soon as it is over, would rapidly fade away for ever.

Our impression of time has very little in common with the laws of physics. Past and future are not on an equal footing. For me, for example, there is no objective "soon": there is only this soon, however long or short it is. There is no "now": there is only this now, of whatever duration. Paradoxically, what each of us knows about time – waiting for a return that is not going to happen; for a love that sooner or later is going to come; in a waiting room for one's turn; the suspense of a castaway at sea or someone trapped under earthquake debris – would be registered by physicists in the space–time relationship that depends on the emotional state of the observer.

Surely, at least once in their life, everyone has closed their eyes, stilled their thoughts and listened to the passage of time in the depths of night? Thoughts seem to be immobilised, indifferent to change. They are moments that can be broken off and suspended, rather than continually chasing after one another. Is this merely an illusion? Pure time has only empty duration, whereas the time we know is memory of the moments that have just gone by or ones which are now remote. No, there is no such thing as pure time because there is no duration without content. Even if our eyelids can screen us from the world around us, patches of light and shade continue to traverse our consciousness. We are immersed in a crowded kaleidoscope of the rhythm being pounded out by the heart, the oscillations of our attention, the images of our thoughts. Our sensation of time is marked by these changes, which are tangible, inconstant, unforeseeable. Can we, then, perceive empty time? Let's close our eyes again, for one whole minute. It's an inconceivably long time! Images from my past life pass before me, the fits of adolescent impatience, the seasons in rapid succession. In just a minute? Yes, because I have looked time in the face, listened to its presence, rejected its illusions.

Our sense of a lasting self

Many years ago Erwin Schrödinger (1958) observed that physics has no theory to account for sensations and perceptions. In order to pursue its research, it has to maintain that such phenomena lie beyond the realm of science. Half a century on there is an even more urgent need for a physics able to recognise the radical difference of time. A physics that helps us to understand how mathematical abstractions, aesthetic preferences, moral judgements and other conscious activities trigger dynamics in our brain that go beyond pure computation. But if our mind works in non-computational terms, then we are in a different domain to the physics we are familiar with. Roger Penrose fully grasped this problem, which concerns first and foremost the radical difference between our perception of the flow of time and the theories of physics.

> A good part of the reason for believing that consciousness is able to influence truth-judgment in a non-algorithmic way stems from consideration of Godel's theorem. If we can see that the role of consciousness is non-algorithmic when forming mathematical judgments, where calculation and rigorous proof constitute such an important factor, then surely we may be persuaded that such a non-algorithmic ingredient could be crucial also for the role of consciousness in more general (non-mathematical) circumstances. (. . .) Whatever algorithm a mathematician might use to establish a mathematical truth, or whatever formal system he might adopt as providing his criterion of truth, there will always be mathematical propositions (. . .) that his algorithm cannot provide an answer for. (Penrose, 1989, p. 538)

Physics denies that internal time is made up of asymmetrical moments of duration and intensity. In order to measure time it has to spatialise it, exteriorise it, adopt symbols or metaphors such as the movement of the hands round the clock face. But clock time does not correspond to the experience of our ego which persists, the succession of thoughts and emotions which follow on from one another incessantly. The ego manifests its liberty – albeit invariably conditioned by or tied to biological constraints – in a movement which unrolls, to use Bergson's metaphor, "like that of a thread on a ball, for our past follows us, it swells incessantly with the present that it picks up on its way" (Bergson, 1955, p. 26)

In his celebrated *On the Phenomenology of the Consciousness of Internal Time* (1893–1917) – the work which can be said to have inaugurated phenomenological research into time – Husserl pronounced some severe strictures on the conceptions of the consciousness of time based on the results, data and combinations of facts or things which can be ordered in time being produced by such researchers in experimental psychology as Helmholtz, Wundt and Fechner. The phenomenological investigation of the structure and consciousness of time, Husserl argued, must deal with determinations which are necessary, logical and formed *a priori*. There is an irreconcilable gap between phenomenology and empirical and experimental rationales. The latter are in the awkward position of having to explain not just the origin of experience and knowledge but also the sequence of temporal events. To the champions of the empirical approach – intent on highlighting only the quantitative aspects of mental data – Husserl pointed out that evidence exists only in the experience that is renewed at each instant (Masullo, 1995). Thus temporality cannot be the sum of segments of experiences but rather something enabling us to go back to the evidence we have acquired, anticipating new testimonies and opening up a horizon of infinite potentialities.

Husserl investigated the concept of time at the point at which it originated and formed. He surprised it, as it were, at the moment of birth, leaving out of account any natural or empirical determination (Husserl, 1893–1917). In its quality as an original source, time is always the onset of something, not the practice of composition. He put forward the hypothesis that consciousness is structured according to temporal modalities and that its dual, indivisible character brings together the modes of relationship of one consciousness with another. Rather than through the connection of one unity to other unities, this synthesis was realised with the unfolding of a unity that is in itself flow. As is well known, this problem led Husserl to introduce the notion of retention: an original point at which the various moments of the flow are joined. There can be no intention that is not joined to a second intention, integrating it and making it possible. In fact consciousness is not internal to the flow, but is itself flow of consciousness: that is, a consciousness which retains the perceived content even when it is no longer perceived.

Each experience, each perception we have, even the most elementary sensation, is a reflex of our being in a continuity, the impression of a permanent flow rather than a transit from one moment to another. Thus the awareness of time is awareness of an extremely changeable rhythm. The stream of our consciousness has an endogenous rhythm of its own (involving vivacity, tiredness, wakefulness, sleep, dream), varying degrees of clarity, its own specific anomalies, and overtly pathological expressions. The awareness of an event – an act, a relationship or whatever in which something that is not homogeneous is perceived as a single unit – arises from an experience that is regarded as unitary with respect to its individual constituent moments. Rather than creating consciousness, these moments occur in it, giving rise to its unity. These are non-linear processes which participate in a multi-level dynamic system, involving complex interactions between brain, body and environment and including the cognitive and conscious acts (Thompson and Varela, 2001).

If it is true that the phenomenon of consciousness is the result of the integrated and distinct activity of the brain, it is also much more than this. While it is always subject to the limits of the body, it goes beyond them, to be transfigured into individual experience in relation to environmental contingencies. This led Varela to make the provocative assertion that "consciousness is not in the head" (Varela, 1996) and that temporality expresses the co-implication of mind and body, not the arithmetical measure of the change.

Consciousness is more than its body. This "more" does not imply any dualism of mind and body but rather an experience that is both unitary and plural. An embodied consciousness has as its correlate temporality itself: a temporality permeated with intentionality, the flow of life which is constituted in and for itself; a temporality, ultimately, which is not synthetic and hence temporal, nor synthetic and at the same time temporal, but "synthetic because temporal" (Husserl, 1893–1917). This is the prime reality – consciousness, in fact – which is always the basic premise because its development derives from the fact that it is "in time" without being "of time".

V

THE NATURAL LOGIC OF MOVEMENT

During the lengthy process of human evolution our ancestors had to adapt to extremely difficult situations. Only rapid choices and timely actions ensured their survival. In order to capture a prey that is moving at 40 km per hour, our forefathers had to anticipate its position in the space of a few milliseconds and position themselves exactly where it was going to be the next instant in an effort of extreme concentration which involved the mind and the whole bodily structure. And this was not all. They also had to prepare the gesture of capture, contracting muscles and overcoming the resistance of bodily weight (Berthoz, 1998). Today the environmental pressures are not the same as in the past, and yet our brain continues to function in the same way. In fact we avoid situations of danger, use our intuition to anticipate the intentions of others, and so on. Our brain is not so much a re-active machine, responding rapidly to environmental solicitations, as a pro-active one that enables us to formulate hypotheses, foresee the consequences of our actions, and even make the first move.

The idea that perception is not just an interpretation of sensorial messages but above all an anticipated simulation of action is not entirely new. As early as 1852 Lotze demonstrated that perception and action were closely related, arguing that the organization of sensorial data is the effect of their integration with information of muscular origin. For Helmholtz (1962), action is more than the outcome of an executive order: it is the ability to confront the sensations with predictions based on motor command. Janet (1935) emphasised the predictive nature of perception: a (retarded) action adapts not only to the stimulus that has provoked it but to all the other potential stimuli generated by the action itself. The modes of perceptive behaviour are characterised by adaptation to a set of purely potential stimuli: when we catch sight of an armchair we have the (illusory) impression of being inert, for we have the characteristic act of the armchair inside us, i.e. a perceptive scheme comprising the act of sitting down in this armchair in a certain fashion. Like a biological simulator, our brain draws on memory and formulates hypotheses of movement, predisposing the actions which are most appropriate to the situation even before it implements them.

Nikola Aleksandrovich Bernstein (1967), one of the fathers of modern physiology, maintained that the planning of a motor act – however it is codified by the nervous system – necessarily implies the recognition of situations that are bound to occur (even though they are not yet even potential). He was one of the first to attempt to go beyond the traditional conception of motor regulation and coordination viewed as a four-phase linear succession: prediction, preparation, performance and verification. He proposed a model based on the cycle of action and perception, with at its core a comparative agent which establishes the so-called "required value" and performs three important functions: (1) identifying the gap between the movement predicted and the one carried out, putting them in correlation; (2) enabling the recognition of an accomplished action, facilitating the passage from one motor sequence to another; and (3) performing an adaptative function, since an unforeseen event can trigger corrective actions to the initial plan of action.

The stringent adaptative requisites have solicited the higher nervous functions to refine, progressively and as rapidly as possible, the capacity for the action's remodulation according to unforeseen events. The body itself – the architecture of the skeleton, the subtle properties of the sensorial receptors, the formidable complexity of the central nervous system – has been designed to ensure the best possible adaptation. These mechanisms have solicited our brain to formulate internal models of the body and the world around us which reflect the over-arching laws of nature and permit the survival of all animals.

Anticipatory representations

In recent years the study of the relationship between perception, action and anticipation has been particularly productive in the world of sport. A large body of evidence has shown that a good level of performance in sport depends not only on technique or the conditional components of motor activity (resistance, force, speed), but above all on so-called "athlete speed": i.e. speed of perception, decision-making, reaction, and above all of anticipation. Moreover, on account of humans' limited capacity for the elaboration of information, it is indispensable to optimise the mental processes. However expert, during performance an athlete is not able to focus on all the external and internal sensorial sources. He or she will have to anticipate the possible actions, making choices and training the attention appropriately, right from the phase of information gathering. In a competition, for example, the necessity for perceptive anticipation – i.e. the ability to make predictions according to information which is only partial or anticipated – derives from the need for rapid reaction and movement times, failing which the motor decisions are likely to be slow and ineffective. By predicting the event the athlete can organize his or her action in advance, choosing the right place and time and completing some typically onerous response selection and programming activities (Abernethy, 1990). This is all the more evident when it is a question of competitive environments in which, on account of the stringent spatial and temporal constraints imposed by the regulations and opponents, being one step ahead can be decisive.

Being able to anticipate perception is above all the prerogative of the experts. A professional skier, for example, does not merely monitor (and if necessary correct) the trajectory of her descent on the basis of the information coming in from her sense organs. In most cases she envisages the route, the various phases and even the possible solutions in case of a mistake. Only occasionally will the brain confront the data coming in from her sensorial receptors with the predictions made in advance. Non-correspondence between the two will lead her to introduce correctives, modifying the angle at which her knees are bent, her speed, and other factors (Berthoz, 1998). The same goes for a tennis player. Without the ability to anticipate, he would systematically miss the ball. In fact several hundred milliseconds elapse between synchronising the muscles to take up a correct posture and the instant in which the racquet reaches the right inclination, during which the ball will have travelled several metres. Hence the need to establish the direction of the ball and its trajectory in advance.

One of the disciplines that has been most closely investigated to understand the functioning of anticipatory mechanisms is karate. During a combat (kumite) – in which two karateki confront each other standing about two metres apart – it is fundamental to achieve the greatest possible postural and motor stability with the minimum expenditure of energy. Thus an expert karateka cannot restrict himself to reacting to unexpected events but has to operate in the future, calling above all on anticipatory actions. Here space and time have very precise limits. On one hand, irrespective of the power put into the performance, the blows have to stop an instant before reaching the adversary's vital parts; on the other, timing is fundamental: even a fraction of a second's delay could have irremediable consequences. To overcome these limits, the karateka has recourse to strategies both of anticipation and compensation. The anticipatory strategies – whose efficacy improves with experience – generate reflex postural responses which stabilise the body, enabling the muscles to contract before the voluntary movement. The probability of success for the motor schemes implemented are directly proportional to the information memorised. This information enables the athlete to develop a sort of internal algorithm which, in a matter of seconds, makes it possible to calculate the value of the variables at stake and to prepare to act on the basis of predictions.

The superior performances of expert athletes also derive from their greater familiarity with what is required. With respect to beginners, they spend much more time imagining themselves in action and studying the performances of their adversaries. These mechanisms can also be observed in soccer. In an experiment performed by Williams and Burwitz (1993) participants were asked to watch on a large screen both sequences of play involving structured attacking schemes (leading to a shot at goal or a pass forwards) and situations which were not structured in which the footballers were involved above all in warm-up activities. After watching them for ten seconds, the participants (some expert, others not) had to recall the positions of the footballers on the computer screen. The non-experts revealed greater margins of error in the structured excerpts. Compensatory strategies come into play, for example, when, following a loss of equilibrium, it is necessary to call on rapid, relatively stereotyped responses, triggered by sensorial stimuli. Of course, these too can improve with experience. In any case, both anticipatory and compensatory responses are set off by information coming from various types of receptors which ensure the automatic maintenance of posture.

While the advantages of the spatio-temporal anticipation mechanisms are perfectly evident, we must also consider the disadvantages that derive from erroneous prediction. If the anticipation mechanisms should produce an inadequate response, the subject will be obliged to inhibit the response and reprogramme the action, paying dearly in terms of time and energy. This error can also be deliberately induced by the opponent. Feints and counterfeints are designed precisely to set up false anticipations, leading to the implementation of motor programmes which are disadvantageous for performance. One can think, for example, of volleyball, in which pretending to play a jump set but actually playing a lob is designed precisely to catch the opposing defence unawares. According to Zaciorskij (1977), the anticipation processes are fundamental both for precision play and for rapid motor decisions. He maintains that 1.5 seconds is the optimum time for beginning an effective anticipatory reaction. In this case too the degree of expertise of the athlete plays a decisive role in the performance's outcome: it is more likely that an expert footballer will formulate a correct prediction and intervene at the right moment, implementing adequate solutions.

Prefiguring

Right from the earliest phases of evolution, the ability to intercept fleeing objects was of decisive importance. In hunting, for example, in order to strike a prey with spear or stone it was fundamental to be able to predict the trajectory of the prey's movements. Whereas to survive attacks from animals (such as a bird of prey swooping down from above), or avoid stones or arrows fired by other human beings, it was necessary to make a proper telemetric assessment so as to anticipate where the strike would come. In situations like these, characterised by stringent temporal constraints, our brain is not able to carry out particularly complicated calculations. It relies on automatic nervous mechanisms based on the relationship between the two dimensions in question: the apparent surface area of the retina and the speed with which the image dilates. If the speed of the object is constant, this relationship can tell us exactly how long there is before contact, allowing us to face up to the strike.

Research into anticipatory skills in sports performances has shown how expert athletes often make use of visual data to sense their opponents' actions. Although coaches invariably advise their charges to 'keep your eye on the ball', expert athletes tend to switch their attention, particularly at critical moments, to different sources of environmental information such as the position of the adversaries, of their team mates, or of objects. In an experiment with baseball going back many years Hubbard and Seng (1954) tried to find out whether, in order to hit the ball, professional batters kept their eyes glued to it throughout its trajectory. They filmed the performances of 29 professional players, and, in spite of some individual discrepancies, results showed conclusively that the expert batters followed the ball with their eyes until it was from 4.5 to 2.4 metres from the bat. The lack of eye or head movements in the last phases of the ball's flight showed that the professional batters possessed an internal representation of the event which enabled them to make effective use of the significant data coming from the pitcher: for example, a bent wrist suggesting a curving ball, an elbow held at right angles pointing to a particularly fast pitch, two fingers on the seam indicating a slider, and so on. It is obvious that batters do not consciously study these indications, but they do act according to this information. After all, in baseball the pitches often reach speeds which are considerably greater than what eye movements are able to follow. So any attempt to follow the ball throughout its trajectory is bound to fail (Gigerenzer, 2009).

But what happens if the ball is in the air, offering a catch? In this case, one of the most commonly used strategies by expert players, even if they are not often conscious of the fact, consists in keeping their eyes on the ball and running, regulating their speed above all by keeping the angle between the eye and the ball constant with respect to the ground. A player who uses this rule has no need to gauge the wind, air resistance, effect of rotation or other variables. All the relevant data are already included in the angle of his observation. The fact that he may have no idea what a differential equation is does not compromise his skill at baseball: things happen beneath the threshold of consciousness which can quite easily be the equivalent of mathematical calculations (Dawkins, 2005).

Among the most effective experiments devised to study the anticipation of moving targets using the eyes there is one that resembles the fairground game of trying to hit and burst balloons which are bobbing up and down on air currents. In the experiment the subject has to keep her eyes fixed on a spot at the centre of a screen. Suddenly another spot appears top right, descending vertically. At this point a beep activated at different moments during this descent instructs the subject to capture the target with a rapid movement of the eyes. The results show that, when the beep sounds, the eyes do not move to the target but towards a point that is further off along its trajectory. This means that, while the eyes were fixed on the spot at the centre of the screen, the brain was assessing the speed of the target as it moved at the periphery of the field of vision, anticipating its future position. In another experiment, researchers looked at the motor differences in the visual anticipation used by footballers as they took a penalty (Savelsbergh et al., 2002). Participants were asked to view films showing sequences of penalty shots as if they were keeping goal, and a control bar was manoeuvred in response to the visual stimuli elicited by the penalty taker. Analysis of the eye movements showed that while the less expert goalkeepers kept their eyes on the player's torso, arms and pelvis for longer, the experts spent more time looking at the posture of the foot making the kick, the supporting foot and the position of the ball at the moment of contact with the foot, revealing in most cases a very accurate capacity of anticipation.

Embodied memories, purposes and action plans

In order to act it is necessary to remember. However, memory is not just a device for re-evoking past events (both internal and external), but also the totality of our corporeal perceptions and senso-motorial schemes and habits. It is no paradox to say that memory carries within it the possibility of actions which have not yet been undertaken. Our present is, at one and the same time, sensation and movement. But, since it is a totality, movement depends on the sensation that is prolonged in action. In this sense, the present constitutes a system of sensations and movements combined: motor sense, in fact. Thanks to the traces of bygone occurrences which lie stored at the bottom of our memory, we are able to anticipate future actions, preparing modes of conduct that will be appropriate for specific purposes. These findings point to the importance of a proactive physiology in the firsthand relationship with the environment, as opposed to the traditional reactive physiology.

There is nothing paradoxical in suggesting the existence of more than five senses (Berthoz, 1998). A perception – as the synthesis of visual, proprioceptive and vestibular information – is always bound to be multisensorial: it depends on mechanisms that are both hierarchical and parallel, and that integrate the information from the sense organs, the signals linked to action and the repertory of prototypes of forms, objects, faces and movements stored in the brain. In its tortuous progress, evolution has established some simplificatory laws of the dynamic, geometrical and kinematic properties of natural movements. All the same, thanks above all to memory, which anticipates the consequences of future action, comparing them with those of past action, perception also reveals predictive capacities. Using his "schema theory" (1975), Schmidt attempted to clarify the relationship between perception, action and memory, highlighting in particular the relations between the prediction of the consequences of the action and the memory of past consequences. His theory is based on two fundamental concepts: the generalised motor programme and the specific motor scheme. The former is a motor pattern stored in the memory representing a class of actions with general, invariable features. Among these we can mention: the sequence of the muscular contractions in a gesture; the temporal structure (i.e. the realization times of the individual movement segments) which remains constant even with variations in the overall movement time; and the relative force, meaning the constant ratio between the forces expressed by the various muscles involved, independently of the degree of overall force. Both variation in and adaptation to the different situational requisites are made possible by changes, during the course of the action, in some parameters such as the selection of specific muscles and the force and duration of the movement.

In the world of sport, for example, the same movement repeated over and over again will never be identical, even if its fundamental structure remains unchanged, confirming the existence of a generalised motor programme. These variations are made possible by the same motor scheme, which is in fact a sort of generalization of concepts (and their inter-relations) deriving from experience, making it possible to identify what is necessary for the performance of a motor programme. In other words, while the generalised motor programme provides the invariable properties of the desired gesture, the motor scheme selects and adapts the specific parameters for the response to the situational needs.

Let us imagine that, prior to taking a penalty, a footballer selects the motor programme and processes the contextual information in the ways he sees best. He will in fact adapt the generalised motor programme to the specific situation, modulating the parameters (time of movement, extent, position of the foot and so on) to the specific needs of the situation (Schmidt and Wrisberg, 2000). The more extensive the variability tested against a specific motor programme, the more precise will be the scheme. In fact, with every variation in the same class, or again as the accuracy of the response feedback increases, the scheme is updated and reinforced, becoming a general rule. Equally, elimination of the specific information solves the problem posed by the quantity of data to be stored.

Schmidt identified two fundamental aspects in schema theory: the recall schema, which permits the introduction of new responses, furnishing the generalised motor programme with the parameters required to perform movements suited to the task; and the recognition schema which, once it is engaged, makes it possible to evaluate the correctness of the movement implemented, comparing the incoming sensorial feedback with what was expected, so as to introduce the necessary corrective measures. This is how the sensorial consequences of the response can be anticipated by means of the confrontation, during and/or after the movement, with the incoming feedback. In this way too information is obtained about the result, and any deviation between the expected and actual sensorial consequences is recognised as an error.

A very similar concept was expressed by Neisser (1976). He argued that perception is a cycle whose fundamental structures comprise anticipatory schemes, i.e. programmes of action that prepare the subject to acquire information which, in turn, will modify the original scheme. In other words, the schemes are being continuously modified by experience, and the information acquired tends to anticipate future choices. For example, if we are using one arm to carry a tray of cocktails and pick up a glass to hand it to someone, we shall keep the tray in equilibrium even if the weight our arm is supporting changes. But if someone helps themselves to a glass, taking us by surprise, there is much less chance of the tray remaining in equilibrium. In this case, in fact, our brain is not able to anticipate the effect of the tray being lightened so as to intervene an instant earlier and modulate the muscular tone in the arm. This anticipatory modality is based on a motor memory (in this case the reference used by the brain is the horizontal state of the tray with respect to gravity).

In performing a motor task the confines between perception and action are not as clear-cut as one might think. If one considers the capacity of elaboration of the cerebral structures, rather than their specific function in the performance of a task, what stands out is not just the role of the frontal lobe in the perception and performance of the action but also that of the basal ganglia in sequencing the movements, language or conception (Boncinelli, 2011). Although they form part of distinct systems, perception and action constitute functions which are integrated.

Natural dynamics

These considerations give even more prominence to the necessity to overcome the hierarchical and pyramidal conception current in the 19th century whereby the motor functions (and hence the body) are subordinated to the higher brain activities. At the origin of abstract modes of behaviour, starting from language, there is the body and its movements. The evolution of some motor modes of behaviour – such as the ability to construct and manipulate instruments – has given rise to an "embodied logic" which has underpinned the subsequent development of the capacity to generate linked movements of the motor and premotor cortex (including the area of Broca), which through the production of gestures and sequences of syllables has imposed itself as the basis of communication. This control of motility, although it preceded language, has contributed to its structuring as an internal motor logic (Oliverio, 2009). Some motor experiences have been of such importance that they have progressively moulded the nervous infrastructures and led to the development of symbols and metaphors used in language, coming to serve as classes of perceptions, behaviour and universal linguistic conventions. Whether we are talking about shaking someone by the hand, writing a letter or whatever, each executive function – thanks to the control of a series of nervous structures and mental processes that process the information – requires behaviours that are oriented to a specific end.

On account of its strategic position and complex relations with the other cortical and subcortical areas – from the working memory (which makes it possible to remember the beginning of a phrase once it has been completed) to behaviours oriented to a specific end (which imply a continuous remodulation of the information with the passage from one action programme to another and the continuous control of the intentional and unintentional effects of our acts) – the frontal cortex is at the heart of the executive functions. More precisely, the prefrontal cortex (in humans this constitutes half of the frontal lobe) is connected to all the other cortical areas and to most of the subcortical structures and is directly or indirectly involved in all the executive functions.

In the light of these complex neural relations, how do we manage to perform actions corresponding to specific purposes? Each executive plan implies hierarchies of significant actions, but can also be part of a more extensive programme of immediate objectives or auxiliary plans which are coherent with the main objective. In any case, these are functions which imply planning and selecting an action, monitoring its performance, and reinforcement associated with the achievement of the given purpose. Ever since the classic research carried out by Leonardo Bianchi (1889) on the effects of the bilateral ablation of the prefrontal cortex in primates, the executive functions of the motor system have always been attributed to the prefrontal lobes. The subtle relationships with behaviour can be recognised precisely in the particular nervous architecture. This can be divided up into prefrontal lateral cortex and prefrontal medial cortex: the former, in its turn, can be subdivided into prefrontal dorso-lateral cortex (which selects the information) and prefrontal ventrolateral cortex (which keeps the stored information); and the latter into anterior cingulate cortex (which identifies the errors of a specific behaviour) and superior frontal gyro (which appears to be involved in the selection and perform-ance of the requisite tasks). These anatomical–functional subdivisions and their implications on behaviour are not always clear-cut. In view of the not infrequent overlapping between anatomical infrastructures and functional dynamics in the definition of the role of the various frontal and prefrontal areas, it is necessary to proceed with great prudence.

This intricate neuronal geography invites us to reconsider the special collaboration between frontal and prefrontal areas. The dynamics of "motor control" seem, to some degree, to run counter to perception. In fact, if perceiving means forming an image of the external world, acting means picturing the intentional consequences of an on-going action. In this sense, the execution of a movement is always linked to a representa-tion of the world on the basis of information made available by the parietal cortex and the hypocampus, this latter structure being involved in many aspects of spatial memory. This information then passes to the premotor cortex, which plans the movement, and finally to the motor cortex, which carries it out. The control and motor performance depend on cortical and subcortical structures, including the basal ganglia which play a role in the control of actions in certain situations and of the moti-vational components of learning. In this scheme, while the cortex and basal ganglia do the planning, the execution of the movement and control over its realization occur in close collaboration with the cerebellum, the red nucleus, the striatum and other subcortical structures.

For almost a century and a half the motor functions have been consid-ered as dependent on the cerebral cortex, which in turn was seen as the site of the highest cognitive activities: rationality, creativity, thought and so on. In reality, even just in representations the activities associated with thought and the motor activities are always closely correlated. Whether it is a question of imagining, planning or acting, the same cerebral areas are always involved. The planning of an action always requires the predic-tion of the consequences, and this type of prediction is invariably the

outcome of activating the action model. In the course of time this intimate connection between thought and motility, which is both
philogenetic and ontogenetic, has produced an archive of extraordinarily
fluid motor repertories. The progressive refining of the relationship
between motor and premotor cortex is at the origin not only of the motor
acts, such as the ability to construct and manipulate objects, but also of
the acquisition of competences by structures like Broca's area and the
basal ganglia, which control the motor aspect of language. This is the case
even if language is not a specific, autonomous system but the product of
a special coordination between various systems and areas of the brain
linked to the representation of objects, perception and indeed corporeal
motility (Oliverio, 2008).

The sentiment of rationality

The tendency to separate the functions of the mind – and above all the
development of a conception which makes the mind superior to the
motor sphere – derives from certain basic philosophical misconceptions
which we would do well to briefly review. While it can be argued that
René Descartes was the instigator of philosophical dualism, it is also true
that he had the merit of casting light on the intimate and immediate relationship which links the mind to our body.

> [It is . . .] by means of those sensations of pain, hunger, thirst etc.,
> that I am not only present to my body as a pilot is present to a ship,
> but that I am very closely *[arctissime]* joined to it and, as it were,
> intermingled with it, so that I compose one thing *[unum quid]* with
> it. For otherwise, when the body is harmed, I, who am nothing
> other than a thinking thing, would not sense pain as a result, but I
> would perceive that harm by the pure intellect, as a pilot perceives
> by sight if something is broken in his ship; and when the body needs
> food or drink, I would understand this fact explicity *[expresse]*, and
> I would not have confused sensations of hunger and thirst.
> (Descartes, Sixth Meditation, AT VII 81/CSM II 56)

In short, mind and body are one and the same thing. We are aware of
what happens in our body, albeit in a different way to how we perceive
external objects. In fact we do not look at our body as we do other things:
we do not have to check the position of our legs, or whether our hands
are in our trouser pockets. We simply know, unlike the unfortunate individuals who, following a vascular accident or some other lesion of the
brain, have lost the sense of bodily movement and their position in space.
To be aware of their movements and their collocation, such people are

obliged to be continually checking the position of their body, just as Descartes' pilot has to tend to his ship.

Apart from the need for a thorough reappraisal of Descartes, there is no doubt that the human nervous system developed in such a way as to coordinate perceptions and movements of the body, and above all to optimise the activities which were essential for survival, such as hunting, mating and bringing up offspring. However paradoxical it may seem, evolution has favoured the development of knowledge for effective action rather than for reflection. William James asked himself whether it is sufficient to have a mere representation of the effects of a movement in order to initiate an action, or if there has to be a further mental event, such as a decision or other analogous phenomenon. He asserted that a movement is always associated with a representation of its consequences. Furthermore, each time a movement is represented, its effectiveness is manifested in the highest degree of intensity as long as it is not hindered by a competing idea in the mind (James, 1890). Like Rudolf Hermann Lotze, James believed that the imagination of a movement activates the same structures that are involved in its execution. Consciousness is always consciousness of an action.

An ancient biological wisdom

The struggle between hunters and hunted has characterised the whole history of evolution. "Survive or succumb" was the harshest law in the times of our ancestors. Understanding in the space of a few seconds whether the rustling in the bushes meant a ravening beast or just a harmless squirrel led our brain, instantaneously, to confront the present with the past and thus to anticipate the future. The question of the instantaneous solution of problems – which involves the relationship between perception and intuition – was studied by the Gestalt psychologists in the first half of the 20th century. They emphasised how, above all in conditions of discriminatory uncertainty, perceptive stratagems closely resemble our intuitive judgements. In fact perceiving also means eliminating ambiguities, choosing one interpretation rather than another: in short, deciding (Berthoz, 2004). And it is thanks to the probabilistic features of perception that we can obtain a unitary representation of the retinal images which are continually changing in form, size, luminosity and other endogenous neurophysiological dynamics. Yet, in spite of these continuous changes, our perception of the world around us is stable and constant. In conditions of uncertainty, in fact, our perceptive system, just like our intuitive judgements, adjusts things, going beyond the information received: I take a gamble on things being one way rather than another. One only has to think of the phenomenon of perceptive constancy, whereby an object or event in the world around us appears to be stable and constant in spite of continuous sensorial variability. This is why we perceive the rectangular shape of a door even as its retinal image varies according to the angle of observation. Our brain merely sees a rectangle that swings on its hinges, even though, as the door opens, it is actually confronted by a sequence of trapezoids.

This is a process of energy saving vis-à-vis the continuous solicitations of perceptive regulation, serving to contrast the risk of inaction. Furthermore, perceptive constancy enables us to perceive objects as if they were endowed with a constant size. When we see a far off person or object, even though the image projected onto the retina is very small, we do not have the impression that they are actually diminished: they are merely far off. This means that, in an automatic and unconscious fashion, our brain has compensated for the variations in size of the retinal image caused by the variations in distance. In practice, perception integrates the representation of the physical world, going beyond the information received, by means of continuous unconscious inferences. Every day we find ourselves seeing partly hidden objects (somebody sitting behind a desk, a dog sitting behind a tree so that we only see its head and tail, or whatever) but perceiving them in their entirety, making sense of our environment. In fact, incomplete or senseless sensorial stimuli are integrated by our brain with mnestic or fantastic material so that the whole perceptive experience is significant. This perception, which goes beyond the sensorial information, is a decision taken by the brain to guarantee a coherent representation of the world.

Intuition: the sixth sense in action

Intuition is not all that different to the perceptive stratagems we have seen above, a form of instinctive and unconscious knowledge which enables us – instead of calling on logical deductive processes – to view and face up to things in a new and often decisive way. Etymologically the term "to intuit" (from the Latin *intuèri*, to look into) indicates a way of looking or knowing using "the mind's eye": the most natural, ancient and universal capacity – an authentic biological wisdom – possessed by human beings (Myers, 2002). Intuition comes into play in situations in which temporal and cognitive–computational constraints prevent us reflecting on or evaluating the data at our disposal. It can save us a great deal of hardship, and it is an extraordinary ally when our very survival is at stake. Indeed, this has been the case since the dawn of time. Being able to decipher rapidly the intentions of whoever you are confronting increases your chances of survival. This explains why often the first instants of an encounter can reveal more than hours of conversation. Besides, in the various cultures the world over, the ability to interpret non-verbal signals is of enormous importance.

In reality, the vast majority of human decisions are intuitive, unconscious and requiring only limited mental input. They enable us to elaborate, rapidly and without any great effort, a considerable amount of information that lies sedimented in our memory, soliciting an immediate and often reliable assessment of the situation on the basis of analogies with past experiences which can reveal unexpected solutions for the problems oppressing us. In any situation in which we have achieved a high degree of experience, an incalculable store of information has been accumulated at the level of "gut instinct". Thus, with just a rapid glance, a chess grandmaster can make the definitive move, or at least the best one possible; an expert entomologist can readily identify the class of the insects she happens to see; or again, a doctor in an emergency situation will recognise an incipient life-threatening risk. In each specific context the ability to distinguish between thousands of different situations and objects is one of the fundamental attributes of the expert and the principal source of intuitions (Simon, 1984).

Over the last twenty years there has been a remarkable surge in the volume of research into the mental mechanisms of instinct, making it difficult, as in other fields, to arrive at a rigorous definition of the term. What is "an intuition": creativity, tacit knowledge, implicit learning and memory, sixth sense, heuristics, emotional intelligence? It really is difficult to say. Intuition has characteristics in common with all these, but also with other definitions. Insight, for example, often considered as synonymous with intuition, regards the sudden comprehension of a problem or a problem-solving strategy, the "Eureka!" moment that arrives after a period of more or less conscious incubation, unblocking the solution to the problem. Intuition takes place almost instantaneously and is made up of a set of emotional and somatic processes, without any role being played (at least apparently) by rational, conscious thought. In fact an intuition almost always has a sensation in the pit of the stomach as its somatic correlate, coming all of a sudden.

But what lies behind all this? One stimulating hypothesis (not without metaphysical overtones) is that a crowd of "cognitive workers" are engaged every day in the subterranean regions of our mind, far from the light of consciousness, elaborating extraordinary quantities of information which involve the implicit memory, heuristics, spontaneous inferences, emotions, creativity and much else besides. Think, for example, of our ability to intuitively recognise a face. Looking at a photo, our brain breaks down the visual information into subcategories (colour, depth and shape) and simultaneously elaborates each aspect, comparing the reconstructed image with ones stored in memory. And so, immediately and apparently effortlessly, amongst thousands of different faces we recognise a person whom we may not have seen for years. True, there is no comparison with the speed at which a computer can match items: the impulses of biological neurons are much slower than those of silicon neurons. But nonetheless our intuitive and unconscious capacities enable us to carry out an incalculable number of actions: catching a ball, converting the bi-dimensional images of the retina into tri-dimensional perceptions, doing up our shoelaces, making a move at chess, and an infinity of other things.

Let us go back for a moment to the situation of driving. We know that when beginners take the wheel, they bring as much attention as possible to the act of driving. They concentrate exclusively on the road, take good care not to talk to other people, and so on. Nonetheless, as time goes on and they acquire experience, the procedures become automatic and their attention is turned to other testing occupations. In reality, things don't always go as they should. How many times, totally occupied by everyday concerns, have we found ourselves at home without any memory of how we got there? And how many times have we missed an exit on the motorway because we were distracted by a phone call or entranced by a song on the radio we hadn't heard for years? Without a precise directive to a specific destination, we would go on automatically performing the tasks we are used to. It is thanks to the efficiency of this automatic, unconscious activity that we can effortlessly complete the routine matters and concentrate on the important things.

Our lives are not regulated merely by conscious choices and actions. Each day we are guided in many of our actions by a sort of automatic pilot. There are days in which, a moment after shutting the front door, we hurriedly check whether we have the keys in our pocket or bag. We don't remember picking them up, even if we did so just a few seconds previously. In the absence of disorders (as in the case of dubitative obsessions) this happens because only the highest cognitive activities attain the level of conscious decisions. Think, for example, of language. Speaking is one of our most important daily actions, and at the same time (apparently) one of the simplest. We utter innumerable word sequences without any effort and perfectly correctly. Just as if, in the engine rooms of our mind, some industrious neuronal workers were intent on composing and decomposing phrases which then come out without the least conscious effort. We do not know how this happens, but it does, and it also happens when we are writing at the computer. The words we see on the screen are the direct expression of the fingers moving over the keyboard, and these in turn are controlled by orders issuing from sophisticated conjunctions of nerves in the midbrain, not from the higher spheres of our mind. In fact, if someone talks to us while we are writing, the fingers don't stop moving, because the indefatigable neuronal workers are capable of terminating the sentence we had begun while we respond to our interlocutor. This phenomenon is all the more surprising in expert pianists, who can quite happily carry on a conversation while their fingers perform a familiar piece. The execution of actions of considerable complexity, like those of someone at the piano, is much more articulated than is suggested by experiments on the programming and performance of simpler movements, contextualised and guided by the executant's skill and judgement (*giudizio*).

All this was already clear to Lotze in the middle of the 19th century:

> We see in writing or piano-playing a great number of very complicated movements following quickly one upon the other, the instigative representations of which remained scarcely a second in consciousness, certainly not long enough to awaken any other volition than the general one of resigning one's self without reserve to the passing over of representation into action. (Lotze, cited in James, 1890, p. 1131)

Without taking into account musical interpretation and the talent of each individual performer, all the components of musical ability derive from a complex interaction between motor learning and temporal elaboration and sequencing, with a crucial role being played by the relations between cortex, cerebellum and basal ganglia.

Look before you leap?

We live in a world which takes it for granted that the quality of a judgement or decision is directly related to the time and effort that go into it. One only has to think of the recommendations parents invariably impart to children: "don't be in a hurry", "think carefully before you make up your mind", "don't make hasty judgements". We are convinced that it is always best, before coming to a conclusion, to assemble all the necessary information and think it over carefully. Nonetheless, as Whitehead claimed a hundred years ago:

> Civilization advances by extending the number of important operations which we can perform without thinking about them. (Whitehead, 1911, p. 61)

Although intuition is based on a very limited amount of information, above all in situations of stress or when time is at a premium, it can rapidly dispel our doubts. This capacity matches our actions to the experiences we have stored in our long-term memory. True, an intuitive thought, devoid of reasoning, can be imprecise and misleading. But we do not only make mistakes when we trust to our intuition. We also err when we think for too long about the actions to take, because we suffocate our gut feelings, depriving ourselves of that particular wisdom. This phenomenon, known as the choking effect, can be seen in particular in the sensorial–motor competence of experts, as for example in an artist or a professional athlete (Baumeister, 1984). Whereas beginners need to focus their attention on each technical detail of their performance, for the professionals, exercising control over a task that has already been automatised may actually be counterproductive (Beilock et al., 2004). In reality, when it comes to giving a performance under psychological pressure (an important début, an audition, an exam), the experts will tend to concentrate more on technical details that are usually performed automatically because they have been acquired as a result of experience. This greater attention to the performance of "step by step" actions is harmful to the skills that have already been interiorised, producing a change in routine which more often than not results in sub-optimal performance. Thus an actor becomes uncertain in speaking his lines, a ballerina loses the fluidity of her movements, a baseball player has more trouble fielding the ball, and so on. In practice the margins of error increase considerably, the performance's natural flow is lost and the grace that accompanies talent vanishes. This is why, at certain levels of experience, we can safely stop thinking.

> The famous pianist Glenn Gould was scheduled to perform Beethoven's opus 109 in Kingston, Ontario. As usual, he started to read through the music first and then play it. Three days before the concert, however, he had a total mental block and was unable to play through a certain passage without seizing up. In desperation, he used an even more intense distraction technique than the experiments with the golfers had. He turned on a vacuum cleaner, a radio, and a television simultaneously, producing so much noise he could no longer hear his own playing. The block vanished. In competitive sports, the same insight can be deliberately used to undermine your opponent psychologically. For instance, while switching courts, ask your tennis opponent what he is doing to make his forehand so brilliant today. You have a good chance of making him think about his swing and weakening his forehand. (Gigerenzer, 2007, p. 36)

There have been a number of experimental investigations in sports confirming that an intentional distraction or a time limit imposed on the execution of a technical gesture does not influence performance, while, on the contrary, the performance is inadequate when the athlete is asked to concentrate on his movements without any time limit. In this sense, the conscious attention, which can only focus on one task at a time, turns to whatever is distracting us without interfering with the motor skills we control best. In an experiment conducted a few years ago, expert and novice golfers had to play a putt either in just three seconds or with no time limit at all (Beilock et al., 2004). In the first case, the novices achieved very poor results, only rarely getting the ball in the hole. The experts, on the other hand, holed the putt more often in three seconds than when they had all the time in the world. The explanation is that the order in which the possible actions came into the players' minds directly reflected their degree of experience: the first was usually better than the second, which in turn was better than the third, and so on. Having more time available to reflect increased the chances of making inefficient choices. If, for example, a golf coach were to advise the expert player to concentrate on the actions to be performed without allowing himself to be distracted by anything, he would begin to make explicit calculations of an enormous number of variables such as the lie of the ball, the distance to the hole, the position of shoulders, hips and feet and so on. Whereas with a beginner exactly the opposite happens: such advice would undoubtedly result in better performance.

Naturally the ability to immediately identify the best choice is not an exclusive prerogative of athletes, as is shown by studies that have been conducted in a whole range of contexts: medical, military, artistic and so on. In the line of research known as naturalistic decision-making – which studies the way in which experts decide on and carry out complex cognitive functions in situations characterised by constraints of various kinds: time pressure, incomplete knowledge of the alternatives, emotional tension, uncertainty, poorly defined objectives, when a lot is at stake – numerous experiments have shown that experts, unlike beginners, have no need to evaluate the pros and cons of each option. Their choices involve a process of recognition of the situation in which the alternatives and potential courses of action are compared on the basis of certain criteria of acceptability (Klein, 1993). For example, if in an emergency situation the commander of a squad of firemen fails to decide in a matter of seconds what has to be done, he risks endangering the lives of many people. All too often, however, the goals are unclear (should the people be brought to safety or the fire be put out rapidly?), the information is uncertain (he has no knowledge of the layout of the building on fire or of what material is inside) and the intervention procedures are not hard and fast (should one use one's imagination to find a way to rescue an injured person trapped in a car crash?). The experts decide by referring rapidly to situations and experiences already encountered in their respective fields. In particular, they intuitively identify which objectives to pursue, the most important indications to be registered and monitored, the possible evolutions of the situation and the relative plans of action (Klein and Crandall, 1995).

When an expert takes a decision, she registers the current situation and acts on the basis of past experiences. The association between the indications registered and the previous experiences enables her to rapidly draw up a possible plan of action. Since experts usually regard the first possibility as the best, it is not necessary to compare all the possible options. In fact the cognitive processing concentrates entirely on how that choice functions with respect to the perceived context. This also permits a greater degree of control over the chosen course of action. If systematic cross-checking between different solutions would generate an ideal solution, investing in a reasonable solution leaves room for the possibility that, rather than being ideal and immutable, it is in fact imperfect and can be modified.

An extremely eloquent example of this is the so-called circumstantial paradigm typical of medical semiotics. Rather than being based on analytical reasoning, it involves an intuitive activity that enables the expert doctor to recognise complaints that could not be diagnosed on the basis of the observation of superficial symptoms which are wholly insignificant to profane eyes. These are forms of knowledge that cannot be formalised or even communicated. No doctor will fully master the art of diagnosis by merely having recourse to the standard diagnostic protocols, for the simple reason that this activity presupposes some imponderable elements such as flair, a keen eye, intuition. Some elements can manifest themselves only to a practised observer endowed with the clinical eye which develops with experience. Being able to make a correct diagnosis with a mere glance, in a short space of time and with few elements to go on, is undoubtedly exclusively the prerogative of the true expert.

VI

THE LOSS OF NATURAL EVIDENCE

I feel I no longer have a body. No, no [. . .] I can still see it. I see my hands, and my body, but it's as if they didn't exist. I can also see my movements, but they are detached from my body. If I look in the mirror I have the impression I'm invisible. My hands do things, but it's like being the captain of a ship of which I am no longer in charge. I speak and the words come out any old how, mechanically, as if I have no control any more. Even the voice doesn't seem to be mine. Perhaps I have died and no one has let me know. My feelings? What can I say about my feelings? What I feel is the absence of any feeling. It's impossible to live like this, day in day out. I pass the time trying to understand what has happened: whether my life is a dream or reality.

MARIA, A PATIENT

During the 20th century philosophers set out to show how common sense and, above all, the words "I", "subject", "we" are illusory constructions. Right from infancy, step by step, we construct a network of connections between what we feel we are, as a result of a representation that is more or less unitary, and our social image. Our identity – the flow of data, signs and events which provides outlines and versions of our personality – appears to us a natural phenomenon. But when subjected to scrupulous phenomenological analysis, the concepts of "I", "subject", "self" are seen to be not single realities but a multiplicity of differentiated features.

What does the word "subject" designate? A name inevitably involves choosing between one statement of reality and another. In identifying with it we allude ourselves that we are subtracting it from the mutability of time. What is that fixed, atemporal image of ourselves that we call "I"? What is its semantic value and how can we come to know it? Again, who am I referring to when I say "I"? And lastly, who is speaking in my voice? If we set aside the reflexes of habit, language and speech, voice and thought appear to be separate realities without any obvious relationship. Beyond the façade of appearances, speaking of oneself implies a paradoxical act, an arduous operation of suture between subjectivisation and desubjectivisation.

In the 20th century the highest poetical and existential evocation of desubjectivation was the life and work of Fernando Pessoa. On 13 January 1935, in reply to a letter from his friend Adolfo Casais Monteiro asking about the origin of his many heteronyms (which the poet attributed to a constant and organic tendency he had to depersonalisation), Pessoa wrote:

> The origin of my heteronyms is basically an aspect of hysteria that exists within me. I don't know whether I am simply a hysteric or if I am more properly a neurasthenic hysteric. I tend toward the second hypothesis, because there are in me evidences of lassitude that hysteria, properly speaking, doesn't encompass in the list of its symptoms. Be that as it may, the mental origin of heteronyms lies in a persistent and organic tendency of mine to depersonalization and simulation. These phenomena - fortunately for me and others - intellectualize themselves. I mean, they don't show up in my practical life, on the surface and in contact with others; they explode inside, and I live with them alone in me . . . . An urging of spirit came upon me, absolutely foreign, for one reason or another, of that which I am, or which I suppose that I am. I spoke to it, immediately, spontaneously, as if it were a certain friend of mine whose name I invented, whose history I adapted, and whose figure, face, build, clothes, and manner, I immediately saw inside of me. And so I contrived and procreated various friends and acquaintances who never existed but whom still today nearly thirty years later I hear, feel, see, repeat: I hear, feel, see and get greetings from them. (Pessoa 1988, pp. 7–9)

Pessoa alludes to the characters who inhabit his mind, separate from the narrator (and different from one another), who alternate and narrate themselves in an extraordinary, unprecedented field of consciousness. His universe is full of figures that are at once real and fantastic, animated by actions running parallel to his formal existence. His subjectivity is split as in a prism: Pessoa becomes Álvaro de Campos, Alberto Caeiro, Ricardo Reis, and still others. Desubjectivisations follow on from new subjectivisations. On 8 March 1914 he observed:

> (. . .) I went up to a high desk, took a sheet of paper and began to write, standing up as I usually do whenever I can. I wrote thirty-

odd poems in one go, in a kind of trance whose nature I cannot define. It was the greatest day of my life and I'll never have another one like it. I started with the title, O Guardador de Rebanhos (The Keeper of Sheep). What followed was the appearance of someone in me, to whom I immediately gave the name of Alberto Caeiro . . . . .So much so, that upon finishing those thirty-odd poems, I immediately took another piece of paper and wrote, also in one go, the six poems that make up *A Chuva Oblíqua* (Oblique Rain), by Fernando Pessoa. Immediately and completely . . . it was the return of Fernando Pessoa, Alberto Caeiro to Fernando Pessoa himself alone. (Pessoa, quoted in Griffin, p. 343)

In this heteronymic kaleidoscope Pessoa transmigrates from himself, only to go back a little later to being who he was before. In him, like the waves of the sea, subjectivisation would give way to desubjectivisation which, to be narrated, requires a re-subjectivisation. The stability of the ego is sorely tested by such different, and at times diametrically opposing, forces. In this vertiginous journey into the core of oneself, who is it that establishes the confines of presence and absence? The self? The unconscious? Pessoa's heteronyms are signs of a flayed existence, not the narration of a medical case history. They testify to the impossibility of a subjective approach to creation and, at the same time, the enigmatic nature of the entity we call "I".

What is this "I"– *punctum crucis* of consciousness, common to reflection, the speech act and poetical creativity – whose nature has never been clarified by anyone? Can we really identify it with the conscious life going on in our mind? If we can, to what is the alienating dissonance between one's identity and the face that figures in a photograph due? It is indeed a curious sensation to be a stranger to myself, but only for myself, not for others. The certainty (of the ego) that drove Descartes to argue that nothing resembles the mind more closely than the mind itself seems to vacillate. The natural evidence of things begins to vanish. The balance between evidence and non- evidence tips in favour of the latter.

The uneasy bond with things

As a rule we do not give any thought to how objects appear to our consciousness. Nor to how conscious acts appear to our reflection. Objects never emerge from their silence. They merely evoke lukewarm passions. And yet it is this immediate rapport with the surface that enables us to become familiar with things, to render our experiences fluid, to make us see eye to eye with others, to establish a continuum between present and past. It is a relationship which is hardly ever compromised, except for variations in vigilance or the outbreak of events with a highly charged emotional content, which may also be independent of external situations. Reflection can only exert a minimal influence on this primary consciousness, showing just how all pervasive it is. That is all. Only the will can act on this archaic experience.

Generally speaking the meaning we project onto things is constantly changing. Things can prove to be more opaque or more transparent, more extraneous or more familiar. Sometimes, however, even what is closest to us can be an obstacle. A change in the relationship with things affects two aspects of everyday life: the stream of consciousness and our harmony with others. It is not a question of making a different value judgement but rather of attributing a different sense to things and other people. In these circumstances the meaning of things distances itself from our consciousness. Subject and object grow further and further apart. New judgements and categories give rise to a different system of values. Our existence gains in profundity but becomes removed from everyday life, which becomes dense with fantastic meanings and categories. The fault line between what the subject feels it is and what it has to be becomes increasingly evident.

Then there are experiences which can tend towards a radical inner metamorphosis (in the schizophrenic sense), deviating the flow of consciousness into obscure byways and suspending every achievement of meaning. In this climate of profound ambivalence, of radical inability to surpass oneself, it is impossible to re-connect and participate in past events. A radical crisis of presence ensues. The instigation of the "as if" modality – i.e. the urge to explain what can no longer be experienced – reveals all the ambiguity of an experience which is incapable of going any further except in a coercive sense. All the psychic energy is concentrated on the "I–world" identification.

Like a marionette

Who doesn't remember the amazement mingled with deep emotion that filled the child Pinocchio when he saw the puppet Pinocchio lying life-less on a chair close by to him? Pinocchio looks at himself, and in so doing he realises he is no longer familiar with his own body, and has lost his usual link with the world of things. Like Pinocchio, many people lose their trust in the things around them, not necessarily because they show psychopathological symptoms. Here we are not recognising a symptom but identifying a phenomenon. Rather than the asymmetry between the content and form of experience, what counts is the lost inherence of the ego to consciousness.

There are perhaps no other human experiences able to reveal the conceptual drama of the unity of the person so starkly as derealization and depersonalization. Certainly, psychiatry and psychology remained ensnared in this dilemma for over a century. Not only do derealization and depersonalization call into question the world's logical structure, transforming the ego into an enigmatic and disconcerting experience; ultimately they show up all the precariousness of rationality's claim to being self-sufficient.

In the debate on psychopathology one often hears the famous and dramatic exclamation – recorded by Jaspers in his *General Psychopathology* (1913) – uttered by a woman from Sandberg at the onset of a delirious fit: "There's something […]. Tell me, what is there? I don't know. But something has happened." It is not my intention to return to a discussion of schizophrenic premonition, which I have dealt with elsewhere (Maldonato, 2001). I just wish to point out how every boundary between the patient and the surrounding world has been dissolved. But if this boundary cannot be designated (whoever is asking cannot be the self, but nor its mirror, which obviously requires the self to exist), who is at the centre of this experience in which everything looms large, posing a terrible threat to the ego? What name can be given to this paradoxical and elusive revelation, this metamorphosis of sense, in which *signifiant* and *signifié* almost come to coincide, obscuring the "who" and "what" of a situation in which nothing has sense any more because everything can have a sense; in which language is a ciphered experience but the code has been lost, and every gesture is an attempt to find refuge in a shared "common sense" before the world ends, before we come face to face with the void?

If the certainty of the subject vacillates – the psychic unity of the individual who institutes truth as the "achievement of meaning" – there are no more explanations, certainties or languages possible. There is only a void, a fantastic aura, a strange atmosphere, progressive and regressive movements of the ego, like currents in the depths of the sea. Outside subjectivity, experience is scattered in a multiplicity of perceptive, affective and cognitive segments. In this sphere of experimentation there is no longer a single reality constituted by the sum of non-egos fused into one artifical ego but another time, another space, another language, which definitively dispel the bond between the ego and the world. The more the boundaries between the ego and the world become uncertain, the more distressful and frenetic the need for self-representation. The more the woman from Sandberg transforms her internal figures into a theatre of shadows and frozen solitudes, the more her inner self becomes a place where nothing is subjective, any more than it is objective.

Falling somewhere between the psychotic condition and the normal human condition, depersonalization reflects the dissolution of the ego as the stable fulcrum of experience, a no man's land where the judgement of reality and the selective power of the perception that endows (and revokes) sense on the world are dissolved. Freed from its ordinary (and artificial) function of integrating the various psychic instances, the ego takes on a polymorphous, original guise. In an inversion of perspective, the experience of the world, constituted up to this point by the reactions of others, becomes charged with potential relationships which are contrasting and equivocal. The actual meaning of objects has been amply superseded. The boundary of the relationship with the other has been abolished. A current bears the ego towards territories which can be sensed although they cannot be traversed. Words like "I", subjectivity and all the other formal devices of language reveal their fundamental inconsistency.

History and stories of depersonalization

Depersonalization was described in the first half of the 19th century as a set of experiences recurring in many psychiatric profiles, characterised by the loss of every sentiment and a sense of unreality vis-à-vis oneself and the world. To designate this latter aspect the term derealization was introduced in the first part of the 20th century. In current international psychiatric classifications, depersonalization is described as a persistent or recurring experience in which subjects feel themselves to be external observers of their mind and their body (as in a dream); while derealization is described as the sensation that the external world has become strange or unreal: as if the size or shape of objects and people have become mechanical and unfamiliar.

The first descriptions of experiences similar to depersonalization can be found in 19th-century medical literature. Griesinger records a letter written by a patient of the famous French psychiatrist Jean-Étienne Dominique Esquirol:

> I continue to suffer constantly; I don't have a moment of comfort, nor experience human sensations. Even though I am surrounded by all that can render life happy and agreeable, in me the faculty of enjoyment and sensation is waiting or have become physical impossibilities. In everything, even in the most tender caresses of my children, I find only bitterness, I cover them with kisses, but there is something between their lips and mine; and this horrid something is between me and the enjoyment of life. My existence is incomplete. The functions and acts of ordinary life, it is true, still remain to me; but in every one of them there is something lacking. That is, the sensation which is proper to them. ... Each of my senses, each part of my proper self is as if it were separated from me

and can no longer afford me any sensation. This impossibility seems to depend upon a void which I feel in the front of my head and to be due to a diminished sensibility over my whole body, for it seems to me that I never actually reach the objects that I touch. I no longer experience the internal feeling of the air when I breathe . . . My eyes see and my spirit perceives, but the sensation of what I see is completely absent. (Griesinger, 1845, p. 157)

Wilhelm Griesinger had often come across similar cases in patients suffering from melancholy. Although they did not manifest any pathology, they complained about experiencing an unbridgeable gap between themselves and things, as if they were cut off from the outside world by a wall. Some years earlier Albertzeller (1838) recorded five patients talking about an almost total lack of feelings: they felt as though they were dead, plunged into a bottomless abyss and with no possibility of seeing daylight ever again. The annotations of another French psychiatrist, Ernest Billod, are also very interesting, describing a patient who reported similar experiences:

She claimed to feel as if she were not dead or alive, as if living in a continuous dream . . . objects [in her environment] looked as if surrounded by a cloud; people seemed to move like shadows, and words seemed to come from a far away world. (Billod, 1847, p. 187)

In reality, the first person to provide a systematic description of these experiences was Maurice Krishaber (1873), who described a total of 38 patients manifesting a mixture of anxiety, asthenia and melancholy. Over a third of them related disconcerting experiences, characterised by the loss of the awareness of reality. Whereas Jules Séglas described the singular case of a patient who lost all consciousness of her body each time she was out walking:

It seems to me as if I am split into two, I lose the awareness of my body, which feels as if it is in front of me, I walk, and I am aware of it but I do not have awareness of my own identity, that it is actually me who is walking. (Séglas, 1895, p. 131)

By the end of the 19th century the hypothesis that experience of the self was only related to the sensorial-perceptive spheres had yielded to a more dynamic hypothesis. Pierre Janet formulated a model of the mind, owing much to the theories of Jackson, which envisaged a psychological organization comprising a complex hierarchy of levels. He considered depersonalization as an aspect of psychoasthenia, a syndrome characterised by a sensation of incompleteness and emptiness which invests perception, motor action, the emotions and the sense of self. It is in fact an authentic pathology of action: "the sensation of void is a problem of action, not of sensations or consciousness" (Janet, 1928, p. 101). The French researcher distinguished between primary and secondary psychic activities: the former include the activities provoked by external stimuli (such as memories), forming a vital impression, while the latter represent an echo of the representations of primary acts and create the illusion of a continuous psychic stream.

> Thousands of resonances constituted by secondary actions fill the spirit during the intervals between external stimuli, and give the impression that it is never empty (. . .) This complex activity links up the [primary] actions brutally determined by the external world, and causes an impression of vitality, or spontaneity, and at the same time of certitude. (Janet, 1928; p. 126)

In these patients there is a tendency to observe themselves, to separate the I–subject from the I–object. Things are wrapped in a sort of "dreamy numbness", a mist, an aura of unreality. The sensation of being inanimate machines is projected onto objects, even the most familiar ones, which lose the quality of being known. And the same sensation invades the patients themselves. Phrases like "as if it wasn't me thinking", "as if my feelings were no longer my own", "as if I'd become an automaton" reflect surprise and disquiet, anguish and apprehension, feelings of being alien and of not belonging. In spite of these metamorphoses of feeling, including feeling part of the world, the critical appraisal of reality generally remains uncompromised, providing a check on the encroachment of the psychosis. The experience of time – in particular, the concordance between then and now – is altered (Callieri & Felici, 1968). It is not unusual for memories themselves to appear alien, as if they no longer concerned the person who experienced them. In any case, the inability to live either in time or outside it is not linked to knowledge of time: rather, it concerns the experience of time. Past, present and future are seen as asymmetric. Feelings of unreality and discontinuity in time are the very essence of depersonalization. Paul Schilder (1935) insisted that depersonalization was typical of psychoses, and it was long believed to be the most frequent of the psychiatric syndromes. While Schilder emphasised the relationship between the corporeal projection and bodily awareness, highlighting the marked analogies between the disorders regarding parts of the body in depersonalised patients, Henry Ey showed how such patients can see and touch their own bodies without ever being convinced that it is their own flesh and bones that are moving. They see their body without recognising it. The progressive estrangement of the body vis-à-vis the self is fostered by the alteration of the emotional sphere, which ensures the maintenance of the bodily image. If the image of our bodies is continually modelled by our sensations and perceptions, the emotional processes constitute the energy and determine that synthesising activity that has been completely lost in this formidable and mysterious experience (Ey, 2005).

VII

THE EXTREMES OF CONSCIOUNESS

> How it is that anything so remarkable as a state of consciousness comes about as the result of irritating nervous tissue, is just as unaccountable as the appearance of Djin when Aladdin rubbed his lamp.
>
> THOMAS HUXLEY

> Language is not a contingent superstructure, nor an anonymous structure of consciousness, but is the structure of consciousness in debate with itself.
>
> HENRY EY

There is a growing consensus among researchers that consciousness originated in a proto-experience which integrated cortical and subcortical dynamics into a temporal structure. At this point of departure intentionality was matched to objects in the real world by means of continuous shifts in perspective (Callieri, 1980). Except in these conditions one could not even imagine those states of attentive and perceptive lucidity, falling between the extremes of sleep and hypervigilance, which enable humans to argue with themselves while fully conscious of their normal and pathological condition. Being the subjective experience of a system in action, consciousness poses serious problems for experimental enquiry, unlike vigilance which can be experimentally investigated with a high degree of approximation.

It has to be said that the ordinary difficulties encountered in talking about consciousness become extraordinary in the domain of alterations of consciousness. Here everything appears more confused and indeterminate. About a century ago Eugen Bleuler believed he could achieve greater clarity by distinguishing the alterations of states of consciousness provoked by organic lesions from the disorders of consciousness due to psychopathological conditions. As we have seen, it was not until the middle of the 20th century that a real advance was made, thanks to the work of Henri Ey. Drawing on an elegant synthesis of the concepts of organization, intentionality and perceptive field, the French psychiatrist described the sphere of consciousness as the horizon within which experience manifests its meaning and the full extent of its momentary, transitory, synchronic breadth. A new appraisal of the conceptual value of this description would give us a better understanding not only of the genealogy, background and stratifications of consciousness, but above all of the evolutionary order of our relational life. In the disorders of consciousness – where neurophysiology intersects with clinical practice in a permanent confrontation between descriptions in the first person and observation in the third person – categories like openness onto the world and the extension and suspension of time are essential factors.

In speaking of a disorder of consciousness it is always useful to pay attention to the presence of qualitative alterations of the sphere of consciousness. Consciousness must not be taken to be synonymous with the sphere of consciousness; nor is it an ordered, circumscribed flow of processes. Being open-ended, consciousness transcends its own sphere of action. Precisely the unity of subjectivity and the world shows how the traditional distinction between the quantitative–categorial levels (attention, vigilance, sleep, coma) and qualitative–dimensional levels (subjective experiences such as sensations, thoughts, emotions) needs to be integrated with an analysis of the hierarchies and different types and degrees of consciousness, whether synchronic (sphere of consciousness) or diachronic (the ego or personality).

Each aspect of our relational life depends on the way in which consciousness integrates and transforms the data received from the environment. However, quite apart from its spontaneous capacity for transformation, consciousness can be strongly modified by our will, as when we concentrate on meditation or withdraw into contemplation. Only the crystal clear perception of our presence – that is, of it being we ourselves who are thinking, knowing, wanting, doing – guarantees a conscious psychic life: precisely what is missing, as we have seen, in those states characterised by sentiments of unreality and loss of familiarity vis-à-vis oneself and the world around, which obscure, like a bank of mist, the outlines of the self, making them indistinct and indeterminate.

Discontinuity of consciousness

The disorders of consciousness are traditionally classed as either quantitative or qualitative. Among the former there are the conditions affecting attention, vigilance and other objectivizable spheres: confusional states, numbness, torpor, coma and cases with an organic basis. Qualitative disorders include those conditions which regard the contents of consciousness, the experience of self and the world around: depersonalization, derealization, dissociative phenomena with a psychogenous basis, oneiric and oneiroid states, confusional and crepuscular states. In reality, this is an artificial distinction. Quite often qualitative disorders are very contiguous to quantitative ones, making it difficult to arrive at a clear demarcation of the two. Of course this is not the place to set about formulating a meticulous (and highly complex) definition of the alterations of consciousness. Nonetheless, in view of their crucial importance in a general consideration of consciousness, we need to outline a general classification. At least four levels of quantitative disorders of consciousness can be identified:

The first level comprises, among others, such clinical expressions as torpor, states of diminished consciousness, hypnoid alterations and others. In these conditions patients still distinguish themselves from the outside world, and fantasy from reality, recognising people and falling asleep normally. It is the first stage on the way to sopor, a sort of pre-coma. These conditions can be triggered by organic causes (cerebral traumas, grave metabolic alterations, tumours) or by the ingestion of alcohol and drugs;

The second level comprises, among others, the oneiric and oneiroid alterations, which involve both quantitative and qualitative associative anomalies, deformation of the appraisal of reality, and the presence of moments of delirium and hallucination. The distinction between reality and fantasy is still partially present. These alterations recur in confusional syndromes with an organic basis (delirium) and in acute phases of schizophrenia and mania.

The third level involves a shrinking of the sphere of consciousness. The onset will be abrupt, the symptomology has a limited duration, and generally the outcome is *restitutio ad integrum*. Patients appear to be totally wrapped up in themselves. They display a progressive inability to integrate temporal and spatial experiences. While there is no incoherence or numbness, they manifest fear, dysphoria, and mystic and ecstatic states. They have little memory of what has occurred. The activity of consciousness involves only a limited area of perceptions, representations, sentiments. The shrinking of the sphere of consciousness has a psychogenous basis and recurs in syndromes such as somatic conversion, post-traumatic stress and prolonged incarceration (Ganser's syndrome). These quantitative disorders can also be caused by epileptic fits, cranial traumas and the ingestion of drugs.

The fourth level comprises, among other things, a confusional state in which the appraisal of reality is absent, there is linguistic incoherence, loss of temporal and spatial orientation, disorganization of language and thought processes, disorders of perception (illusions, hallucinations), alterations of the sleep-waking rhythm. It recurs in such cases as delirium or in acute and chronic organic confusional syndromes, traumas, dysmetabolic conditions, tumors and toxic states.

The qualitative disorders of consciousness include phenomena of derealization and depersonalization, disorders of dissociative identity (formerly known as multiple personality), psychogenous amnesia, somatic conversion syndrome, somatoform disorders, post-traumatic stress syndrome, acute psychoses and others. They can develop through medical causes (mostly following on from cerebral alterations) or psychic causes as the expression of a defence that intervenes in extreme situations (trauma) and unconscious conflicts that serve to contain a distress that cannot be organized in any other way.

In historical terms the psychopathological study of consciousness was of great importance. The formal features identified by Jaspers (1913) are still fundamental:

Sense of activity. Relational life is underpinned by an original activity which cannot be reduced to any other thing. The ego is conscious of thinking, acting and so on. This sense of the individual's presence is lacking in states of depersonalization, where instead there is a radical perceptive estrangement, automatism of the will, a prevailing feeling of the absence of personal sentiments;

Consciousness of uniqueness. I am a single whole at any given moment. The fact that the stability of the ego is beyond doubt, for all its extreme variability, is demonstrated by dissociations of personality;

Consciousness of identity. I am what I was yesterday through the flux of time;

Consciousness of the ego as opposed to the outside world and others. This aspect fully displays the unrepeatable originality of relational life.

The harmonious development of these features – which according to Jaspers are at the basis of consciousness – is strongly altered by the ingestion of narcotic and psychedelic substances (cannabinoids and psilocybin, mescaline and lysergic acid, as well as more recent forms) and is manifested in phenomena such as the diffusion of thought (patients have the impression that their thoughts are projected onto the environment) and the sensation of fearful change with the onset of schizophrenia, feeling at the mercy of obscure forces, under hypnosis and other states.

Whether these are identified as quantitative or qualitative disorders, their psychopathological study must always go hand in hand with analysis of the evolution and dissolution of the relationship between cortical and subcortical structures. For example, lesions of the ARAS, like the dysfunction of both cerebral hemispheres, can cause quantitative alterations of the state of consciousness. Alternatively, cortical lesions, in the absence of a bilateral dysfunction, produce modifications of the contents of consciousness matching their functional specialization.

A recent work (Baars et al., 2003) compares the major physiopathological states linked with the absence of consciousness (deep sleep, coma/vegetative state, general anaesthesis, loss of consciousness during an epileptic fit). In particular it is shown how these states, although caused by a varied aetiopathogenesis, all share a series of objectivizable elements: regular electroencephalographic activity, a noticeable diminution of the metabolism in the frontoparietal regions, a generalised blockage of both cortico-cortical and talamo-cortical functional connections, and a state of "non respondence". These effects of destructuring enable us to understand better some aspects of the temporal structure of consciousness and the related neural processes. For example, there are patients who can sleep well, be attentive and converse agreeably while showing no sign of consciousness disorders or altered syntony. And yet these are patients who often know very little of what they should know: where they are or where they have just come from. They often make mistakes, get lost easily, do not know the date or time or how old they are. Even in the state of full vigilance they are incapable (or only partially capable) of retrieving lost information.

Although the debate on these highly sensitive issues is making great strides in the scientific community, in standard clinical practice alterations of the state of consciousness are still defined using the concepts of vigilance and consciousness. For example, if a patient involuntarily shuts their eyes, this is automatically classed as a withdrawal of consciousness from the world. If in a coma consciousness has disappeared and, in the most serious cases, the vital functions (such as breathing) have to be mechanically assisted, in the vegetative state the patient alternates periods when the eyes are opened and closed, often in correspondence with the sleep–waking cycles. Unlike in a coma, in the vegetative state there may be an unmotivated motor and facial mimicry activity. Although there are a large number of factors to be taken into consideration, before drifting into the vegetative state patients usually spend some weeks in the state of coma, after which the risk of non-return becomes all too tragically probable.

In addition to the vegetative state there are states of minimal consciousness, and here the terminological and clinical situation becomes even more confused. The diagnostic criteria for this rather "all embracing" syndrome, characterised by severe alterations of consciousness, are different from those regarding the vegetative state.

Consciousness is only minimally and discontinuously present. Patients appear to be able to interact, spontaneously or in response to precise stimulations, in an almost congruous way, albeit intermittently, with the outside world. However, their actions will not include the execution of complex tasks or last any length of time. In fact these two clinical conditions have notable elements in common, and they have been brought together in a clinical spectrum labelled "low level neurological state", making it possible to dispense with such dated concepts as apallic syndrome, vigil coma and others.

ENVOI

For every one of us, consciousness is a primary, immediate, permanent fact, the core of life itself. Why, then, if we start thinking about it, do we have the impression that we are always far from forming any definitive picture, any hard and fast truth, however partial? The enthusiastic essays and the disproved hypotheses, the doubts and the certainties, the reservations and the renunciations we have come across in this brief journey reveal not only the fragility of unilateral conceptions but also the difficulties of a pluridimensional interpretation. The intractable attitude of determinists and materialists who seem to be immunised against the use of even one psychological term is offset by the sense of proportion shown by such pioneers as Jackson, Sherrington, Ey, Penfield, Eccles and many others who devoted their lives to throwing light on the intricate labyrinths of the brain. In view of their exemplary experience as researchers, it would have been wholly coherent for them to identify with a materialist perspective. Why didn't they do so? Simply because they were not interested in coming up with reassuring shortcuts, and above all because they had no ambition to attain to visions of the world.

In his later years Eccles declared that one day the roots of consciousness would be found in nature. To date, he argued, hypotheses had only dealt with some of the links existing between specific cerebral events and psychic experiences, not the essence of this relationship. Dissatisfied with the predominant approaches, the Australian evoked the existence of a system in which matter and energy were combined, reflected in the dynamic patterns of the cortical neuronal activity in some states of consciousness. This system would allow the brain to connect to the mind like a highly sensitive detector. The contact with the mind would involve a critical point of excitation of no apparent significance located somewhere in the brain. In support of this hypothesis Eccles recalled that the ablation of significant parts of the cerebral cortex or the presence of particular physio-pathological activities (an alpha rhythm or a convulsion) do not suspend consciousness. He was perfectly conscious of the risk that the dualism implicit in his hypothesis could come to dominate its reception. The answer he gave was neither elusive nor diplomatic: there exists a mental entity, he claimed, coinciding with man's very nature, which manifests itself through a physical organ in a particular state of activity essential to this manifestation.

The reality may in fact be very different to how Eccles imagined it. And yet we cannot help asking: has science really helped us to gain an understanding of consciousness, or is this destined to remain an inaccessible mystery for ever? There are still no convincing arguments for the existence of a mental activity outside the brain. Naturally, this does not mean that religious meditation or philosophical research do not have a sacrosanct right to investigate consciousness. On the contrary! The task of researchers is to explore its structure in the scope of their relational lives. This remains the sense and the limit of a science of consciousness, in spite of the enormous extension of the semantic field which this term has undergone in the course of time.

The study of the biological bases for consciousness has shown how physics is incapable of providing credible solutions to this problem. If it is true that *qualia* are qualitative phenomena determined by complex integrative states; it is no less true that, in their rapid mutability, they can generate new states and new conscious forms. Some time ago, Edelman asserted that *qualia* are not caused by neural states, any more than the haemoglobin spectrum is caused by the structure of the protein, and that maintaining the contrary would be to go against the very laws of physics. The lack of means to describe the enormous quantity of interactions between neuronal structures and qualitative experiences in detail prevents us from going any further in research.

This explanatory shortfall does not authorise us, of course, to postulate the existence of an inaccessible *sancta sanctorum*. Both physics and biology arise out of human experience. Man is part of nature and wholly immersed in it. A project to naturalise consciousness – attempting to ground our relational life and human action in biology – has to recognise a special role for complexity and for the irreversibility and historical contingency of our phenomenalistic experience. The fact that to date scientists' attempts to explain consciousness have fallen wide of the mark is not in fact serious: there is time for everyone to try a different track. Science is also a powerful instrument for identifying errors and exercising a rational control over illusions while nonetheless being aware that, for all its rigour, it will never be immune to error nor able to tackle the questions that assail it in isolation. The recognition of its limits does not obscure the fascination and marvel which nature elicits in scientists. Like explorers of unknown regions, scientists concentrate on the radical questions that generate surprise and astonishment, the same sentiments which our ancestors felt thousands of years ago when confronted with phenomena to which they could give no name. Marvelling at the existence of things, just like a child discovering the world, opens up the path to knowledge and causes us to exclaim "How extraordinary this all is!" It is the mystery which makes us look beyond the surface of things and interrogate the world.

Richard Feynman has spoken memorably about the mystery and astonishment of the vocation of research. To him the last word:

> Poets say science takes away from the beauty of the stars - mere globs of gas atoms. Nothing is "mere". I too can see the stars on a desert night, and feel them. But do I see less or more? The vastness of the heavens stretches my imagination — stuck on this carousel my little eye can catch one-million-year-old light. A vast pattern — of which I am a part (. . .) What is the pattern or the meaning or the why? It does not do harm to the mystery to know a little more about it. For far more marvelous is the truth than any artists of the past imagined! (Feynman, 2011, p. 59)

REFERENCES

Abernethy B. (1990), "Anticipation in squash: Differences in advance cue utilisation between expert and novice players", *Journal of Sports Sciences*, 8, 17–34.

Baars B.J. (1988), *A Cognitive Theory of Consciousness*, Cambridge University Press, Cambridge.

Baars B.J. (1997), *In the Theater of Consciousness: The Workspace of the Mind*, Oxford University Press, New York.

Baars B.J., Ramsøy T.Z., Laureys S. (2003), "Brain, conscious experience and the observing self", *Trends in Neurosciences*, 26 (12), 671–675.

Bauer G. (1990), "Der teufel steckt im Detail", *Fussballtraining*, vol. 11, 3–7.

Baumeister R.F. (1984), "Choking under pressure: Self-consciousness and paradoxical effects of incentives on skillful 'performance'", *Journal of Personality and Social Psychology*, 46, 610–620.

Beilock S.L., Berenthal B.I., McCoy A.M, Carr T.H. (2004), "Haste does not always make waste: expertise, direction of attention, and speed versus accuracy in performing sensorimotor skills", *Psychonomic Bulletin & Review*, 11, 373–379.

Bencivenga, E. (2008), *Anime danzanti*, Aragno, Torino.

Bergson H. (1889), trad. it. *Saggio sui dati immediati della coscienza*, Raffaello Cortina, Milano, 2002.

Bernstein N. A. (1967), *The Coordination and Regulation of Movement*, Pergamon Press, New York.

Berthoz A. (1998), trad. it. *Il senso del movimento*, McGraw-Hill, Milano.

Berthoz A. (2004), trad. it. *La scienza della decisione*, Codice Edizioni, Torino.

Bianchi L. (1889), *Semiotica delle malattie del sistema nervoso*, Vallardi, Milano.

Billod E. (1847), "Maladies de la volonté", *Annales Médico-Psychologiques*, 10, 187.

Bleuler M. (1961), "Bewusstseinstorungen in der Psichiatrie". In H. Staub, H. Thoelen, *Bewusstseinstorungen*, Thieme, Stuttgart.

Block N., Fodor J. A. (1972), "What psychological states are not", *Philosophical Review*, 81, 159–181.

Block N. (1978), "Troubles with Functionalism" in *Minnesota Studies in the*

Philosophy of Science, vol. 9, University of Minnesota Press: Minneapolis, pp. 261–325.

Blumenberg H. (1985), trad. it. *Naufragio con spettatore*, Il Mulino, Bologna.

Boncinelli E. (2011), *La vita della nostra mente*, Laterza, Roma-Bari.

Boring E.G. (1970), "Attention: Research and beliefs concerning the concept in scientific psychology before 1930". In D.I. Mostofsky D.J. (a cura di), *Attention: Contemporary Theory and Analysis*, Appleton-Century-Crofts, New York.

Callieri B. (1980), "L'accesso fenomenologico alla coscienza in psichiatria, I. Tra l'empirico e il trascendentale", *Rivista di Biologia*, 73, 170–190.

Callieri B., Felici F. (1968), "La depersonalizzazione. Psicopatologia e clinica", *Rivista sperimentale di freniatria*, 93, 2, 573–751.

Chalmers D. (1996), *The Conscious Mind: in Search of a Fundamental Theory*, Oxford University Press, New York.

Changeux J-P. (1998), trad. it. *L'uomo neuronale*, Feltrinelli, Milano.

Crick F. (1994), *The Astonishing Hypothesis*, Scribner, New York.

Crick F., Koch C. (1992), "The Problem of Consciousness", *Scientific American*, September, 111–117.

Dawkins R. (2005), trad. it. *Il gene egoista*, Mondadori, Milano.

Descartes R. (1641), trad. it. *Meditazioni sulla filosofia prima (a cura di G. Brianese)*, Mursia, Milano, 1994.

Dehaene S., Kerszberg M., Changeux J.-P. (1998), "A neuronal model of a global workspace in effortful cognitive tasks", *Neurobiology*, 95 (24), 14529–14534.

Dennett D.C. (1991), *Consciousness Explained*, Little Brown & Co., Boston.

Edelman G. (1989), trad. it. *The Remembered Present: A Biological Theory of Consciousness*, Basic Books, New York.

Edelman G.M. (1992), trad. it. *Sulla materia della mente*, Adelphi, Milano, 1993.

Edelman G.M., G. Tonini (2000), trad. it. *Un universo di coscienza. Come la materia diventa immaginazione*, Einaudi, Torino.

Ey H. (1963), *La conscience*, PUF, Paris.

Ey H. (1967), *Manuel de Psychiatrie*, Masson, Paris.

Ey H. (1978), *Conscioussnes: A Phenomenological Study of Being Conscious and Becoming Conscious*, Indiana University Press, Bloomington.

Ey H. (2005), *Le déchiffrement de l'inconscient; Travaux psychanalytiques (texte de 1964)*, L'Harmattan, Paris.

Feynman R.P. (2000), trad. it. *Sei pezzi facili*, Adelphi, Milano.

Fodor J. (1983), trad. it. *La mente modulare*, Il Mulino, Bologna.

Fodor J. (2001), trad. it. *La mente non funziona così. La portata e i limiti della psicologia computazionale*, Laterza, Roma-Bari.

Fraisse P. (1987), "Temporal structuration of cognitive processes: discussion", intervento al convegno Strutturazione temporale dei processi cognitivi. In O. Belardinelli (a cura di), *Comunicazioni scientifiche di Psicologia Generale*, 15, Bulzoni, Roma.

Freud S. (1886–1895), trad. it. *Opere. 1. Studi sull'isteria e altri scritti*, Boringhieri, Torino, 1977.

Frith C. (2002), "Attention to action and awareness of other minds", *Consciousness and Cognition*, 11, 481–487.

Gazzaniga M. S. (1997), *La mente della natura*, Garzanti, Milano.

Gigerenzer G. (2009), trad. it. *Decisioni intuitive*, Raffaello Cortina, Milano.

Goodwin F. K., Jamison K. R. (1990), *Maniac Depressive Disorder*, Oxford University Press, Oxford.

Griesinger W. (1845), *Pathologie und therapie der psychischen krankheiten*, Adolf Krabbe Verlag, Stuttgart.

Haggard P., Clark S., Kalogeras, J. (2002), "Voluntary action and conscious awareness", *Nature Neuroscience*, 5 (4), 382–385.

Helmholtz H. (von) (1962), *Treatise on Physiological Optics*, Dover, New York.

Hubbard A.W., Seng C.N. (1954), "Effects of stress contrasts on certain articulatory parameters", *Phonetica*, 24, 23–44.

Husserl E. (1931), trad. it. *Meditazioni cartesiane. Con l'aggiunta dei discorsi parigini*, Bompiani, Milano, 1963.

Husserl E. (1893–1917), "Lezioni sulla coscienza interna del tempo". In E. Husserl, trad. it. *Per la fenomenologia della coscienza interna del tempo (1893–1917) (a cura di A. Marini)*, Franco Angeli, Milano, 1981.

Husserl E. (1923–1924), *Erste Philosophie (1923/1924)*, Martinus Nijhoff, Dordrecht.

Ishai A. (2002), "Streams of Consciousness", *Journal of Cognitive Neuroscience*, 14 (6), 832–833.

Jackendoff R. (1987), *Consciousness and the Computational Mind*, MIT Press, Cambridge, Massachussetts.

Jackson F. (1982), "Epiphenomenal Qualia", *Philosophical Quaterly*, 32, 127–136.

Jackson F. (1986), "What Mary didn't know", *Journal of Philosophy*, 83, 291–295.

Jackson J.H. (1884), "The Croonian Lectures on Evolution and Dissolution of the Nervous System", *The British Medical Journal*, 1 (1214), 660–663.

James W. (1890), trad. it. *Principi di psicologia*, Società Editrice Libraria, Milano, 1901.

James W. (1904), "Does 'consciousness' exist?", *Journal of Philosophy, Psychology, and Scientific Methods*, 1, 477–491.

James W. (1909), trad. it. *Un universo pluralistico*, Marietti, Casale Monferrato, 1973.

James W. (1912), *Essays in Radical Empiricism*, Longmans, Green and Co., New York.

Janet P. (1903), *Les obsessions et la psychasthénie*, Félix Alcan, Paris.

Janet P. (1928), *L'évolution de la mémoire et de la notion du temps*, Chahine, Paris.

Janet P. (1935), *Les Débuts de l'intelligence*, Flammarion, Paris.

Jaspers K. (1913), trad. it. *Psicopatologia generale*, Il Pensiero Scientifico, Roma, 1964.

Kandel E.R. (2006), *In search of Memory: The Emergence of a New Science of Mind*, Norton, New York.

Klein G.A. (1993), "Recognition-primed decisions". In W.B. Rouse (ed.), *Advances in man-machine systems research*, JAI Press, Greenwich.

Klein G.A., & Crandall B.W. (1995), "The role of mental simulation in naturalistic decision making". In P. Hancock, J. Floch, J. Caird & K. Vincente (eds.) *Local Application of the Ecological Approach to Human-Machine Systems* (vol. 2, pp. 324–358). Erlbaum, Hillsdale, NJ.

Kotchoubey B. (2007), "Event-related potentials predict the outcome of the vegetative state", *Editorial, Clinical Neurophysiology*, 118 (3), 477–479.

Kripke S.A. (1971), "Identity and Necessity". In M. Munitz (ed.), *Identity and Individuation*, New York University Press, New York.

Krishaber M. (1873), *De la Neuropathie Cerebro-Cardiaque*, Masson, Paris.

Långsjö J.W., Alkire M.T., Kaskinoro K., Hayama H., Maksimow A., Kaisti K.K., Aalto S., Aantaa R., Jääskeläinen S.K., Revonsuo A., Scheinin H. (2012), "Returning from Oblivion: Imaging the neural core of consciousness", *The Journal of Neuroscience*, 32 (14), 4935–4943.

Laureys S., Owen A.M., Schiff N.D. (2004), "Brain function in coma, vegetative state, and related disorders", *The Lancet Neurology*, 3, 537–546.

Le Van Quyen M., Adam C., Lachaux J-P., Martinerie J., Baulac M., Renault B., Varela F. J. (1997), "Temporal patterns in human epileptic activity are modulated by perceptual discriminations", *NeuroReport*, 8, 1703–10.

Libet B. (2007), trad. it. *Mind Time. Il fattore temporale nella coscienza*, Raffaello Cortina, Milano.

Lloyd D. (2002), "Functional MRI and the Study of Human Consciousness", *Journal of Cognitive Neuroscience*, 14, 818–831.

Lotze R.H. (1852), *Medizinische Psychologie oder Physiologie der Seele*, Weidemann, Leipzig.

Maldonato M. (2001), "Saggio introduttivo". In B. Callieri, *Quando vince l'ombra. Problemi di psicopatologia clinica*, Edizioni Universitarie Romane, Roma.

Mancia M. (1994), *Neurofisiologia*, Raffaello Cortina, Milano.

Masullo A. (1995), *Il tempo e la grazia. Per un'etica attiva della salvezza*, Donzelli, Roma.

McGinn C. (1991), *The Problem of Consciousness*. Blackwell, Oxford.

Midorikawa A., Kawamura M., Takaya R. (2006), "A disconnection syndrome due to agenesis of the corpus callosum: disturbance of unilateral synchronization", *Cortex*, 42, 356–65.

Miller J.G. (1950), *Unconsciousness*, John Wiley & Sons, New York.

Moruzzi G., Magoun H. (1949), "Brain stem reticular formation and activation of the EEG", *EEG Clin. Neurophysiol*, 1, 455, 1949.

Myers D.G. (2002), *Intuition: its Power and Perils*, Yale University Press, London.

Nagel T. (1974), "What is it like to be a bat?", *The Philosophical Review*, Vol. 83, N. 4, pp. 435–450.

Neisser U. (1976), *Cognition and Reality*, W.H. Freeman, San Francisco.

Oliverio A. (2008), *Geografia della mente: territori cerebrali e comportamenti umani*, Raffaello Cortina, Milano.

Oliverio A. (2009), *La vita nascosta del cervello*, Giunti, Firenze.

Parasuraman R., Davies D.R. (1984), *Varieties of Attention*, Academic press, Orlando.

Penrose R. (1992), trad. it. *La mente nuova dell'imperatore*, Rizzoli, Milano.

Pessoa F. (1923–1935), *Correspondência. 1923–1935*, edição Manuela Parreira da Silva, Assírio & Alvim, Lisboa, 1999.

Plum F., Posner J.B. (2000), trad. it. *Stupor e coma*, SEU, Roma.

Proust M. (1922), *Swann's Way* (Translator: C. K. Scott Moncrieff). London, Chatto and Windus.

Ramachandran V. (2004), *The emerging mind*, Profile Books, London.

Ribot T. (1881), *Les maladies de la mémoire*, L'Harmattan, Paris (2005).

Ribot T. (1882), *Les Maladies de la volonté*, Félix Alcan Editeur, Paris, (1909).

Ribot T. (1885), *Les Maladies de la personnalité*, Félix Alcan Editeur, Paris (1889).

Savelsbergh G.J.P., Williams A.M., Van der Kamp J., Ward P. (2002), "Visual search, anticipation and expertise in soccer goalkeepers", *Journal of Sports Sciences*, 20, 279–287.

Schilder P. (1935), trad. it. *Immagine di sé e schema corporeo*, Franco Angeli, Milano, 1973.

Schmidt R.A. (1975), "A schema theory of discrete motor skill learning", *Psychological Review*, 82, 225–260.

Schmidt R.A. (1982), *Motor control and learning: a behavioral emphasis*, Human Kinetics Publishers, Champaign, Illinois.

Schmidt R.A., Wrisberg C.A. (2000), Motor learning and performance (2nd ed.), Human Kinetics Publishers, Champaign, Illinois.

Schrödinger E. (1958), *Mind and Matter*, Cambridge University Press, Cambridge.

Séglas J. (1887–1894), *Leçons cliniques sur les maladies mentales et nerveuses*, Asselin e Houseau, Paris, 1895.

Simon H.A. (1984), trad. it. *La ragione nelle vicende umane*, il Mulino, Bologna.

Squire L.R., Kandel E.R. (1999), *Memory: from mind to molecules*, Scientific American Library, New York.

Thompson E., Varela F. J. (2001), "Radical embodiment: neural dynamics and consciousness", *Trends in Cognitive Sciences*, 5, 418–425.

Varela F.J. (1996), "Neurophenomenology: a methodological remedy for the hard problem", *Journal of Consciousness Studies*, 3 (4), 330–50.

Walshe F.M.R. (1957), "The brain-stem conceived as the 'highest level' of function in the nervous system, with particular reference to the 'automatic apparatus' of Carpenter (1850) and to the 'centrencephalic integrating system' of Penfield", *Brain*, 80, 510–539.

Wilkinson I., Lennox G. (2007), trad. it. *Manuale di neurologia*, Minerva Medica, Torino.

Williams A.M., Burwitz L. (1993), "Advance cue utilization in soccer". In T. Reilly, A.M. Williams, (eds.), *Science and Football II*, Routledge, London.

Winson J. (1986), *Brain and Psyche: The Biology of the Unconscious*, Garden City, New York.

Zaciorskij V.M. (1977), *Die körperlichen eigenschaften des sportlers*, Bartels & Wernitz, Berlin, Frankfurt, Munchen.

Zeki S., Bartels A. (1998a), "Toward a theory of visual consciousness", *Consciousness and Cognition*, 8 (2), 225–259.

Zeki, S., Bartels A. (1998b), "The asynchrony of consciousness", Proceedings of the Royal Society of London, 265, 1583–1585.

Zeller A. (1838), "Uber einige Hauptpunkte in der Erforschung und Heilung der Seelenstörungen", *Zeitschrift fur Beurtheilung und beilung der krankhafte Seelenzustände*, 1, 512–569.

INDEX